Pass the ABSITE!

Pass the ABSITE!

Rafael Azuaje, M.D.
Department of Surgery
Indiana University
School of Medicine
Indianapolis, Indiana

Carlos Vieira, M.D.
Department of Surgery
Indiana University
School of Medicine
Indianapolis, Indiana

SAUNDERS
An Imprint of Elsevier Science
Philadelphia London New York St. Louis Sydney Toronto

SAUNDERS
An Imprint of Elsevier Science

The Curtis Center
Independence Square West
Philadelphia, Pennsylvania 19106

PASS THE ABSITE! ISBN 0–7216–1021–8

Library of Congress Cataloging-in-Publication Data
Azuaje, Rafael.
Pass the ABSITE! / Rafael Azuaje, Carlos Vieira.
p. ; cm.
ISBN 0–7216–1021–8
1. Surgery–Examinations, questions, etc. 2. Surgery, Operative–Examinations, questions, etc. 3. Surgery, Operative–Examinations–Study guides. I. Title: Pass the American Board of Surgery In-Training Examination. II. Vieira, Carlos. III. Title. [DNLM: 1. Surgical Procedures, Operative–Examination Questions. 2. Specialty Boards.
WO 18.2 A997p 2003]
RD28.A1 A98 2003
617′.0076–dc21 2002075770

CE MVY
Publishing Director—Surgery: Andrew Stevenson
Acquisitions Editor: Joseph Rusko
Project Manager: Jodi Kaye
Book Designer: Gene Harris

Printed in the United States of America.
Last digit is the print number: 9 8 7 6 5 4 3 2 1

To Reina and Ernesto (CAV)

To my wife, M Alice, and my daughter Caroline, for making everything possible. (REA)

Notice

Contributors

Rafael Azuaje, M.D.
Department of Surgery, Indiana University,
School of Medicine, Indianapolis, Indiana

David Brandli, M.D.
Department of Urology, Indiana University,
School of Medicine, Indianapolis, Indiana
Urology

Patrick Connolly, M.D.
Department of Neurosurgery, Indiana University,
School of Medicine, Indianapolis, Indiana
Neurosurgery for the General Surgeon

Virgilio George, M.D.
Department of Surgery, Indiana University,
School of Medicine, Indianapolis, Indiana
Anesthesia for the General Surgeon

William Hoffmann, M.D.
Department of Otolaryngology, Indiana University,
School of Medicine, Indianapolis, Indiana
Otolaryngology (Ear, Nose, Throat)

Carlos Vieira, M.D.
Department of Surgery, Indiana University,
School of Medicine, Indianapolis, Indiana

Preface

Preparing for the Surgery Boards can be stressful and difficult to accomplish. There are many subjects in general surgery and surgical specialties that require thorough review in a limited time.

This book provides a rapid review for surgeons and general surgery residents preparing for the Surgery Boards. Our goal was to gather high-yield information and present it in an easy-to-read question-and-answer format, followed by a detailed explanation that also covers related topics. Actually, most of the questions involve several different concepts in one single question. This will prepare you for the "real test" and help you assess your areas of strength and weakness. We have included many "test question" facts, as well as those that we find useful in surgical clinical practice. The chapters have been organized by subject, both in basic and clinical science. The last section covers the surgical specialties. In addition, up-to-date references have been included to facilitate further study in specific areas.

The clinical information presented in this book should be used as a guide only. Proper diagnosis and treatment should be individualized to each patient. It is *not* designed to be a comprehensive text or an isolated source, but a time-saving aid to be used when preparing for the test.

We hope that this book will help you increase your board scores. We are sure that you will enjoy it. Good luck on your exams!

RAFAEL AZUAJE, M.D.
CARLOS VIEIRA, M.D.

Acknowledgments: *Pass the ABSITE!* was made possible by the contribution of many surgery residents, who helped us select the most relevant study material for the in-service examination and for the General Surgery Boards. We also express our sincere gratitude to **Sara Highbaugh**, who helped us organize this book. Finally, we wish to thank **Jay L. Grosfeld, M.D.** and **James A. Madura, M.D.** for their full support and guidance during our surgical training.

Contents

PART ONE: *Basic Science*

PART TWO: *Clinical Science*

PART THREE: *High-Yield Facts*

Disclaimer: The American Board of Surgery In-Training Examination is a test administered by the American Board of Surgery. ABSITE is a trademark of the American Board of Surgery, Inc, which neither sponsors nor endorses this book.

PART ONE

Basic Science

Surgical Principles, Homeostasis, and Physiology

QUESTIONS

1. Many trauma centers in the United States now use ultrasound in the evaluation of abdominal trauma. The four-view trauma examination (or focused abdominal sonogram for trauma—FAST) performed by nonradiologists has the following characteristics, except:
   a. It is performed with a 3.5-MHz probe.
   b. The probe is placed in the right midaxillary line between the 11th and 12th ribs to identify Morison's pouch.
   c. The left upper quadrant is evaluated with the probe in the left anterior axillary line between the 10th and 11th ribs.
   d. In experienced hands, ultrasound imaging has been associated with a negative laparotomy rate of 5%, comparing favorably with both computed tomography and diagnostic peritoneal lavage.
   e. The amount of fluid in the abdomen reliably detected by ultrasound imaging is somewhere between 200 and 650 mL.

2. Our understanding of the molecules that mediate cell–cell adhesion and adhesion of cells to proteins within the extracellular matrix has progressed rapidly in recent years. In regard to these molecules (cellular adhesion

molecules [CAMs]), which of the following statements is NOT true:

a. The β_2-integrins are expressed exclusively on platelets and are critical for platelet migration to sites of inflammation.
b. There are four groups: integrins, cadherins, members of the immunoglobulin superfamily, and selectins.
c. The enhanced cell surface expression of selectins is associated with slowing and rolling of leukocytes along the endothelial cell wall.
d. Cadherins play a central part in the maintenance of tight intracellular contact, as seen in the zone adherens and the desmosomes.
e. Intracellular CAM-1 (ICAM-1) and vascular CAM-1 (VCAM-1) exhibit increased cell surface expression in response to tumor necrosis factor α, lipopolysaccharide, and thrombin.

3. Which segment of the gastrointestinal tract absorbs the majority of the water intake?
   a. Jejunum
   b. Ileum
   c. Ascending colon
   d. Transverse colon
   e. Sigmoid colon

4. Oxygen delivery is dependent on all the factors listed below, except:
   a. Cardiac output
   b. Hemoglobin
   c. Oxygen saturation
   d. Arterial oxygen pressure
   e. Metabolic acidosis

5. A 70-kg, 45-year-old white man presents with hemoptysis, loss of weight, and low-grade

fever. A chest radiograph reveals a cavitary lesion on the apex of the right lung. On his second day of hospitalization, the patient experiences altered mental status. Serum sodium level is 115 mEq/L. The total amount of sodium needed to correct this isovolemic hyponatremia is:

a. 480 mEq
b. 540 mEq
c. 630 mEq
d. 750 mEq
e. 800 mEq

6. With an intestinal anastomosis, which is the strongest layer of the bowel wall that supports it?
   a. Mucosa
   b. Muscularis mucosa
   c. Submucosa
   d. Muscular layer
   e. Serosa

7. What is the fluid turnover rate of the normal pleural space per day?
   a. Less than 200 mL
   b. 200 to 600 mL
   c. 600 to 1000 mL
   d. 1000 to 1400 mL
   e. 1400 to 1800 mL

8. Which of the following conditions does not present with splenomegaly?
   a. Felty syndrome
   b. Spherocytosis
   c. Idiopathic thrombocytopenic purpura
   d. Myeloid metaplasia
   e. Hodgkin disease (nodular sclerosis type)

9. A 42-year-old woman comes to the emergency department complaining of shortness of breath.

Physical examination and chest radiography show a large left pleural effusion. The laboratory results from the thoracocentesis specimen shows: cloudy appearance, a white blood cell count of 13,000/mm^3, a red blood cell count of 1000/mm^3, low glucose, 3.5 g/dL of protein, a 0.93 lactate dehydrogenase ratio, and a density of 1020. All of the following may cause this problem except:

a. Pleural metastasis from breast cancer
b. Tuberculosis
c. Acute pancreatitis
d. Systemic lupus erythematosus
e. Glomerulopathy

10. What is the most common cause of unilateral chylothorax?
    a. Surgical trauma
    b. Pancoast tumor
    c. Superior vena cava thrombosis
    d. Left subclavian vein line placement
    e. Lymphoma

11. Which of the following is the most sensitive diagnostic method for acute renal failure?
    a. Glomerular filtration rate
    b. Serum creatinine
    c. Fractional excretion of sodium (FeNa)
    d. Creatinine clearance
    e. Ultrasonography

12. Which of the following tissues does not have a vascular lymphatic system?
    a. Thymus
    b. Liver
    c. Skeletal muscle
    d. Esophagus
    e. Adrenal gland

13. Regarding hepatorenal syndrome, which of the following statements is correct?
    a. A renal biopsy usually reveals acute tubular necrosis.
    b. Patients present with moderate to severe hypernatremia.
    c. Urinary sodium is usually less than 5 mmol/L.
    d. Urinary osmolarity is less than plasma osmolarity.
    e. Liver and kidney transplantation is the optimal treatment.

14. Regarding inguinal and abdominal wall hernias, which one of the following statements is incorrect?
    a. The most common hernia in females is the indirect inguinal hernia.
    b. A sliding hernia on the right usually involves the cecum.
    c. Attempts to reduce a strangulated hernia should be carried out after the patient is sedated.
    d. Repair of an inguinal hernia in infants should not be delayed and consists only of high ligation of the hernia sac.
    e. Grynfeltt hernia is a lumbar hernia localized between the 12th rib and internal oblique muscle.

15. The gastroduodenal artery is an important branch of the:
    a. Left gastric artery
    b. Right gastric artery
    c. Common hepatic artery
    d. Superior mesenteric artery
    e. Splenic artery

16. A 55-year-old man with hypertension and hypercholesterolemia comes to the clinic with symptoms of intermittent claudication of the lower extremities. You decide to prescribe lovastatin to reduce his cholesterol levels. What is the mechanism of action of lovastatin?
    a. Increase 7-α-hydroxylase activity
    b. Inhibit hydroxymethylglutaryl-CoA reductase
    c. Increase lipoprotein lipase
    d. Inhibit hormone-sensitive lipase
    e. Increase lecithin cholesterol acyltransferase
17. Glucagon is an important peptide hormone. Regarding its actions, which statement is incorrect?
    a. Glucagon promotes glycogenolysis, gluconeogenesis, and ureogenesis.
    b. Glucagon promotes insulin secretion.
    c. The primary target for glucagon action is liver and skeletal muscle.
    d. Its action is mediated by increase of cyclic guanosine monophosphate.
    e. Insulin, hyperglycemia, and somatostatin inhibit secretion of glucagon.
18. Regarding parathyroid cancer, which one of the following statements is true?
    a. It is a frequent cause of hyperparathyroidism.
    b. Most patients present with hypercalcemia and a palpable mass.
    c. The histopathologic criteria to differentiate parathyroid adenoma and parathyroid carcinoma are well defined.
    d. It is associated with multiple endocrine neoplasia type 1.
    e. Localizing studies are mandatory before neck exploration.

ANSWERS

1. ULTRASOUND FOR SURGEONS/PERITONEAL ANATOMY: correct answer c

Ultrasound is rapidly becoming a useful and valuable tool for trauma surgeons in the United States. This user-friendly technology has unique qualities: rapidity, portability, safety, and noninvasiveness. An ultrasound examination (FAST) provides a survey of the dependent regions of the pericardial sac and abdomen for the detection of fluid (blood). It can be done in about 2.5 minutes. After initial stabilization, the sonogram is performed with a 3.5-MHz probe during the secondary survey with the patient in the supine position. Water-soluble, warmed, hypoallergenic ultrasound transmission gel is applied in four specific areas: pericardial area, right upper abdominal quadrant, left upper abdominal quadrant, and pouch of Douglas. The transducer is oriented for sagittal sections and positioned in the subxiphoid region to identify the heart and to examine for blood in the pericardial sac. The probe is then placed in the right midaxillary line between the 11th and 12th ribs to identify the sagittal section (the liver, kidney, and diaphragm) and to examine for blood in Morison's pouch (between the right kidney and liver). With the probe positioned in the left posterior axillary line between the 10th and 11th ribs, the spleen and kidney are then visualized. Fluid (blood) is sought in the splenorenal recess and in the subdiaphragmatic space. The probe is then placed 4 cm superior to the symphysis pubis, directed for coronal sections, and moved inferiorly toward the symphysis pubis in a sweeping fashion.[1]

In experienced hands, ultrasound has been associated with a negative laparotomy rate of 5%, comparing favorably with both computed tomography and diagnostic peritoneal lavage.

Peritoneal Anatomy. The abdomen of a supine patient consists of seven dependent spaces: right and left supramesocolic, right and left paracolic gutter, right inframesocolic, and pelvic cul-de-sac. In reality, however, fluid within the abdomen of a supine patient usually flows to the supramesocolic compartments or the pelvis, almost regardless of the source. This is particularly relevant because nearly all trauma patients are transported and evaluated in the supine position. The pelvis (rectovesicular pouch in men, rectouterine pouch in women) is the most dependent overall intraperitoneal space (supine), and the right hepatorenal fossa (the Morison pouch) is the most dependent supramesocolic location. Pelvic fluid spills over the sacral promontory and ascends the right paracolic gutter to collect in the Morison pouch. The phrenocolic ligament prevents spread down the left paracolic gutter, and the fluid from the left supramesocolic area (spleen) spreads over the lumbar spine to the Morison pouch and down the right paracolic gutter to the pelvis.[2]

The amount of fluid in the abdomen reliably detected by ultrasound is between 200 and 650 mL and is influenced by patient position. As a point of reference, a diagnostic peritoneal lavage (DPL) count of 100,000 red blood cells/mm^3 reflects 20 mL of intra-abdominal blood mixed into 1 L of lavage fluid. Computed tomography reportedly detects 100 to 250 mL of intra-abdominal fluid.

2. CELL ADHESION MOLECULES: correct answer a

Specific cell surface proteins are involved in mediating adhesion of cells to each other and of cells to extracellular matrix structures. The ability to characterize CAMs at the molecular level has made possible the classification of these molecules into several discrete groups that include integrins, cadherins, members of the immunoglobulin superfamily, and selectins. These proteins are involved in events such as the recruitment of platelets to the site of plug formation and establishment of the epithelial layer of the intestinal lining, the binding of a neutrophil or lymphocyte to the endothelial layer, and the adhesion of cells to extracellular matrix proteins, as occurs with adhesion of cells to the basement membrane along the vascular wall. The cadherins represent a family of adhesion molecules that include “classic” cadherins as well as subfamilies of structurally related proteins. They play a critical role in processes such as embryonic development, formation of the epithelial layers of the skin and intestine, and axonal formation in the nervous system. The classic cadherins were among the earliest identified in this family and comprise the N, P, R, B, and E cadherins. Ca^{2+} is critical to its function and serves to maintain the structural integrity of the protein. Cadherins play a central part in the maintenance of tight intracellular contact, as occurs in the zone adherens and the desmosomes.

The integrins are a set of cell surface adhesion molecules that regulate cell–cell and cell–extracellular matrix protein interactions. The β_1-integrins contribute to tissue organization by binding to molecules both in the extracellular matrix within many tissues and in the basement membranes found in muscle, the nervous system, epithelial tissue, and endothelium. β_1-Integrins also have a role in lymphocyte homing and leukocyte migration. The β_2-integrins are expressed exclusively on leukocytes and are critical for leukocyte migration to sites of inflammation. The β_3-integrins have been identified on platelets and cells of the megakaryoblastoid lineage. Members of this subfamily play a key role in platelet activation and thrombosis. α_5-, β_3-Integrins and β_1-integrins have been identified on breast cancer cells and may be involved in the metastatic process, and several histopathologic studies have established a correlation between α_6-, β_4-integrin expression and tumor progression. The major ligands for the integrins fall into two categories: cell surface molecules that are members of the immunoglobulin supergene family (such as intracellular adhesion molecules [ICAM-1, ICAM-2], vascular cell adhesion molecule [VCAM-1], or mucosal addressin cell adhesion molecule [MAdCAM-1]) and a variety of large extracellular matrix proteins (such as fibronectin, vitronectin, fibrinogen, and complement component iC3b).

In the immune system, immunoglobulin supergene family members play a critical role in cellular adhesion. Key members include the ICAMs, of which there are now five members, VCAM-1, and the peripheral addressin, MAdCAM-1. These proteins serve as ligands for the integrins. ICAM-1 and VCAM-1 exhibit increased cell surface expression in response to tumor necrosis factor α, lipopolysaccharide, and thrombin. Such agents as interferon-α and interleukin-4 regulate the expression of either ICAM-1 or VCAM-1, respectively.

The selectin family of proteins forms the newest family of adhesion molecules. At present, it is a small family composed of L, E, and P selectin. The selectins are expressed in low levels on the cell surface. On activation of cells with inflammatory stimuli, P selectin is recruited to the cell surface from storage in Weibel-Palade bodies. E selectin is synthesized and transported to the cell surface upon exposure to a range of inflammatory mediators. L selectin is present on the cell surface of leukocytes. In addition, L selectin is shed from the cell surface into the circulation. The enhanced cell surface expression of selectins is associated with slowing and rolling of leukocytes along the endothelial cell wall.[3]

3. GASTROINTESTINAL PHYSIOLOGY: correct answer c

Although the entire length of the colon (approximately 135 cm) has the capacity to absorb water and specific electrolytes, most of this absorptive capacity occurs in the ascending colon.[4]

4. OXYGEN DELIVERY: correct answer e

Before we define oxygen delivery, we must understand what oxygen content is. The oxygen concentration in the arterial blood, known as oxygen content ($Caco_2$), is dependent on oxygen saturation, hemoglobin, and arterial Pao_2 as described in the following equation:

$$Caco_2 = (1.34 \times Hb \times Sao_2) + (0.003 \times Pao_2)$$

The first term of the equation states that each gram of hemoglobin binds to 1.34 cc oxygen when fully saturated with oxygen.

The second term of the equation describes the contribution of the oxygen dissolved in plasma. At a normal body temperature of 37°C, the solubility of the oxygen in plasma is 0.028 cc/L/mm Hg. In order to express the concentration in cc/100 cc, the solubility coefficient is divided by 10, creating the second term of the equation: $0.003 \times Pao_2$.

It is interesting that changes in hemoglobin have a major impact on arterial oxygenation compared with changes in Pao_2.

Oxygen delivery ($\dot{D}o_2$) is the product of cardiac output (CO) and arterial oxygen content ($Caco_2$).

The normal range for oxygen delivery is 520 to 570 cc/min/m^2.[5, 6]

5. HYPONATREMIA: correct answer c

The management of hyponatremia is determined by the state of the extracellular compartment and the patient's symptoms. Patients with symptoms have to be treated more aggressively, with hypertonic saline (3% NaCl).

The rate of rise in plasma sodium should not exceed 0.5 mEq/L/hr, and the final plasma sodium concentration should not exceed 130 mEq/L initially.

The amount of sodium to be given is calculated based on the sodium deficit:

$$\text{Sodium deficit (mEq)} = \text{Normal total body water} \times (130 - \text{Current P Na})$$

The normal body water (in liters) is 60% of the body weight in kilograms, so in our scenario:

$$0.6 \times 70 \times (130 - 115) = 630 \text{ mEq}$$

Because 3% of sodium chloride contains 513 mEq of sodium/L, the volume of hypertonic saline to correct the hyponatremia will be 630 ÷ 513 = 1.22 L. Using a maximal rate of 0.5 mEq/L/hr, the sodium deficit should be corrected over 30 hours.[6–8]

6. ANATOMY: correct answer c

The strongest layer of the bowel wall that supports an intestinal anastomosis is the submucosa because of its greater amount of collagen fibers.[9]

7. ANATOMY: correct answer c

The pleura produces 600 to 1000 mL of fluid per day, and an equal amount is reabsorbed. Pleural fluid is formed primarily from the parietal pleura, and part of its turnover depends on the same Starling forces that govern vascular and interstitial fluid exchange. The subpleural lymphatics represent the major pathway for liquid and solute drainage. The lymphatics can absorb up to 20 times more fluid than is normally formed.

8. SPLENOMEGALY: correct answer c

Idiopathic thrombocytopenic purpura (ITP) is an autoimmune disease wherein IgG antiplatelet antibodies destroy the circulating platelets. The spleen plays a major role in removing previously sensitized platelets. ITP occurs mostly in adults, particularly in women of childbearing age. The disease presents usually with a history of easy bruising, hematomas to minimal trauma, gum hemorrhage, or even hematuria or melena. Low platelet counts and increased bleeding time are strongly suggestive of ITP.

The spleen is of normal size, and histologically there is congestion of the sinusoids and enlargement of the follicles. Acute ITP has an excellent prognosis in children, with a full recovery in around 80% of patients. In adults, the initial therapy is a steroid trial for 2 months. If the patient does not respond to the initial steroid treatment, splenectomy is indicated (~80% response rate).[10]

Felty syndrome refers to the triad of rheumatoid arthritis, splenomegaly, and neutropenia. Steroids and splenectomy have been used to treat the neutropenia. Hodgkin lymphoma can present with splenomegaly. Splenectomy is considered in cases of stage I or stage II Hodgkin disease during staging laparotomy or for palliation when the total platelet number severely decreases.

Spherocytosis is an autosomal dominant disease wherein spectrin, the major protein membrane of the erythrocytes, is absent. Clinical features include splenomegaly, jaundice, and anemia. Treatment is splenectomy. If gallstones are present during the operation, cholecystectomy should be performed. Myeloid metaplasia is a panproliferative process manifested by increased connective tissue proliferation of the bone marrow, liver, spleen, and lymph nodes. The treatment usually is directed at the anemia and splenomegaly. Although splenectomy does not change the course of the disease, it is indicated in symptomatic (left upper quadrant pain), anemic, or thrombocytopenic patients.[11]

9. EXUDATES: correct answer e

The classic characteristics of an exudate are:

Color: cloudy to tan
White blood cell count >10,000/mm^3
Red blood cell count >10,000/mm^3
Glucose low
Protein >3.0 g/dL
Specific gravity >1016
Lactate dehydrogenase ratio >0.6
pH <7.2
Culture may be positive (empyema).
Cytology may be positive (malignant).

Malignancy (primary and metastatic), infection (specific or nonspecific), infarction, sympathetic disease (pancreatitis, subphrenic abscess), trauma, and collagen-vascular disease (rheumatoid arthritis, systemic lupus erythematosus) are common causes of exudative pleural effusions.

All glomerulopathies involve protein loss causing a decrease in the plasmatic oncotic pressure, leading to a transudate-type pleural effusion.[11]

10. CHYLOTHORAX: correct answer a

Leakage of lymphatic fluid (chyle) from the thoracic duct produces a characteristic milky effusion called *chylothorax*. The most common cause is iatrogenic injury of the thoracic duct, most frequently after distal esophagectomy or procedures that involve dissection in the lower left cervical region at the confluence of the left subclavian and left internal jugular veins and mediastinal lymph node dissections for testicular cancers. Traumatic chylothorax is almost always unilateral, usually on the left side. The most common nontraumatic chylothoraxes are related to venous hypertension in the brachiocephalic system (superior vena cava thrombosis). The least common variety of nontraumatic chylothoraxes are lymphomas and lung tumors (Pancoast) caused by a neoplastic obstruction of the lymphatic channels.[11]

11. RENAL PHYSIOLOGY: correct answer c

Fractional excretion of sodium (FeNa): The gold standard for the diagnosis of acute renal failure is renal biopsy. Renal biopsy usually is not performed in patients with acute renal failure because of its invasiveness. FeNa is considered the best noninvasive test to diagnose and differentiate prerenal azotemia, renal azotemia, and postrenal failure.

Prerenal failure is associated with loss of volume and can be due to dehydration, hypoproteinemia with third spacing, blood loss, or septic or cardiogenic shock.

Intrarenal causes are those involving intrinsic injury to the kidneys and can be produced by medications (most commons are aminoglycosides, cyclosporine, nonsteroidal anti-inflammatory drugs), toxins (endotoxins), radiopaque contrast material, and pigmented nephropathy (myoglobin released after crush injuries, hemolysis, burns, and major operative procedures).

Postrenal causes include ureteral obstruction (stones, trauma, surgical injury), bladder obstruction (drugs, nerve injury, or tumors), and urethral obstruction (trauma, benign prostatic obstruction, and malignancy).[12]

To calculate the FeNa, spot measurements of urine sodium and creatinine should be performed. In prerenal azotemia, the kidneys try to preserve sodium, resulting in a low urinary sodium and a low fractional excretion of sodium. FeNa is calculated using the following formula:

$$\text{FeNa} = (\text{urinary Na} \times \text{plasma creatinine}) \div (\text{plasma Na} \times \text{urine creatinine})$$

Table 1–1 summarizes the useful parameters for substances detectable in urine used in the diagnosis of acute renal failure.

12. LYMPH VASCULAR SYSTEM: correct answer a

Lymphatics are found in all tissues except the central nervous system, cartilage, bone and bone marrow, thymus, teeth, and placenta.[13]

TABLE 1—1

Useful Parameters for Substances Detectable in Urine Used in the Diagnosis of Acute Renal Failure

	Prerenal	Intrarenal	Postrenal
Urine osmolality (mEq)	>500	<350	Variable
Urine/plasma osmolality	>1.25	<1.1	Variable
Urine/plasma creatinine	>40	<20	<20
Urine Na	<20	>40	>40
FeNa	<1	>3	>3

13. HEPATORENAL SYNDROME (HRS): correct answer c

HRS is a serious and almost always deadly complication in patients with end-stage liver disease. HRS seems to be a final stage of the complex hemodynamic derangements associated with portal hypertension and ascites, which include systemic vasodilatation, hypovolemia, and hyperkinetic circulation. Indeed, the major features of HRS are azotemia, hyponatremia, and hypotension. The kidneys are structurally intact, and results of kidney ultrasonography, pyelography, urinalysis, and even kidney biopsies are all normal. In fact, the kidneys of patients with this syndrome have been used for transplantation with a good outcome. It is important to differentiate and exclude other causes, especially prerenal azotemia. The urine sodium concentration is less than 5 mmol/L, a concentration lower than occurring in prerenal azotemia. The urine sediment is unremarkable. The criteria for HRS have been reviewed by the International Ascites Club and is summarized as follows:

Major Criteria:

a. Chronic or acute liver failure with advanced hepatic failure and portal hypertension
b. Low glomerular filtration rate, indicated by a serum creatinine value >1.5 mg/dL or creatinine clearance <40 mL/min
c. Absence of treatment with nephrotoxic drugs, shock, infection, or significant fluid losses
d. No sustained improvement in renal function after diuretic withdrawal and volume expansion with 1.5 L isotonic saline
e. Proteinuria <500 mg/dL and no ultrasonographic evidence of obstruction or parenchymal renal disease

Additional Criteria:

a. Urine volume <500 mL/day
b. Urine sodium <10 mEq/L
c. Urine osmolality greater than plasma osmolality
d. Urine red blood cell level <50 per high-power field
e. Serum sodium concentration <130 mEq/L

In the absence of clearly reversible causes, the prognosis of HRS is dismal. Orthotopic liver transplantation remains the ultimate treatment of choice. When liver transplantation is successful, full kidney recovery is expected.[14–16]

14. HERNIAS: correct answer c

The most common hernia in males and females is the indirect inguinal hernia. Femoral hernias are more common in females than in males. A sliding hernia occurs when the visceral peritoneum of an organ makes up part of the wall of the hernia sac. A sliding hernia usually involves the cecum on the right or the sigmoid colon on the left. In females, ovaries or fallopian tubes, or both, can be involved.

Strangulated hernias should not be reduced. Reduction should be performed in the operating room after inspection of the contents of the hernia sac. Incarcerated hernias should be reduced after appropriate patient sedation.[9]

Repair of an inguinal hernia in children should not be delayed and consists of a high ligation of the hernia sac. Conversely, umbilical hernia repair can be delayed until the patient is 4 years old and hydrocele until age 1 year.

Grynfeltt hernia is a lumbar hernia between the last rib and the internal oblique muscle. *Petit hernia* is a lower lumbar hernia whose boundaries are the iliac crest, latissimus dorsi muscle, and external oblique muscle.[17] *Spigelian hernia* occurs at the lateral border of the rectus at the level of the linea semicircularis. *Littre hernia* occurs when a Meckel diverticulum is the only component of the hernia sac. *Richter hernia* is considered a noncircumferential incarceration of the antimesenteric border of the intestines into the hernia sac.

15. GASTRIC ANATOMY: correct answer c

The gastroduodenal artery is an important branch of the common hepatic artery. This artery branches at the level of the head of the pancreas into anterior and posterior superior pancreaticoduodenal arteries. Another important branch of the gastroduodenal artery is the gastroepiploic artery, which supplies blood to the greater curvature of the stomach together with the left gastroepiploic artery, a branch of the splenic artery.[17, 18]

16. ANTIHYPERLIPIDEMIC DRUGS: correct answer b

Lovastatin is one of the three drugs (pravastatin, simvastatin) that inhibit HMG-CoA reductase, the rate-limiting enzyme in the synthesis of cholesterol. Compensatory mechanisms cause decrease in low-density lipoproteins and triglycerides and inhibit hepatic synthesis of very-low-density lipoproteins.[19]

17. PANCREATIC PHYSIOLOGY: correct answer d

Glucagon is a catabolic hormone secreted by alpha cells of the pancreatic islets. Glucagon is considered a “fasting hormone” and promotes the delivery of substrates to peripheral tissues by:

Increasing liver gluconeogenesis
Increasing liver glycogenolysis

Increasing liver ketogenesis
Increasing ureogenesis

Its action is mediated by the increase of cyclic adenosine monophosphate (cAMP). cAMP activates protein kinase A, which by catalyzing phosphorylation alters the activity of enzymes such as glycogen phosphorylase and acetyl CoA carboxylase.

Glucagon action is stimulated by hypoglycemia, amino acids (especially arginine and lysine), and an increase of sympathetic and parasympathetic outflow.

Glucagon action is inhibited by hyperglycemia, insulin secretion, and somatostatin. Interestingly enough, glucagon is one of the most important hormones that promote insulin secretion.[20]

18. PARATHYROID CARCINOMA: correct answer b

Parathyroid cancer is not a frequent cause of hyperparathyroidism, accounting for less than 1% of cases. Approximately 85% of patients with parathyroid cancer present with abnormal calcium and parathyroid hormone levels. The histologic criteria for malignancy are poorly defined. History, physical examination, and evidence of local or distant invasion may play a key role in differentiating between malignant and benign disease.

Multiple endocrine neoplasia types 1 and 2 are associated with hyperparathyroidism due to parathyroid hyperplasia or parathyroid adenoma.

Localizing studies, including computed tomography of the neck, magnetic resonance imaging, venous sampling, and nuclear medicine imaging are not mandatory before neck exploration. The sensitivity of radiologic studies still ranges from 70% to 85% and should be ordered only when the diagnosis of parathyroid disease is in doubt.[7, 20]

Quick Answers

1. C	7. C	13. C
2. A	8. C	14. C
3. C	9. E	15. C
4. E	10. A	16. B
5. C	11. C	17. D
6. C	12. A	18. C

REFERENCES

1. Simon B, Snoey E: Ultrasound in Emergency and Ambulatory Medicine, 1st ed. St. Louis: Mosby, 1997, pp 151–189.
2. Staren E: Ultrasound for the Surgeon, 1st ed. Philadelphia: Lippincott-Raven, 1997, pp 123–136.
3. Petrzzelli L, et al. Structure and Function of Cell Adhesion Molecules. Am J Med 106:467–476, 1999.
4. Sabiston D: The Biological Basis of Modern Surgical Practice, 15th ed. Philadelphia: WB Saunders, 1997, p 975.
5. Marino PL: The ICU Book, 2nd ed. Baltimore: Williams & Wilkins, 1998.
6. Miller RD: Anesthesia, 5th ed. Philadelphia: Churchill Livingstone, 2000.
7. Townsend CM, Beauchamp RD, Evers BM, Mattox K: Sabiston Textbook of Surgery, 16th ed. Philadelphia: WB Saunders, 2001.
8. Bone RC, George RB, Reynolds HY, et al: Pulmonary & Critical Care Medicine. St. Louis: CV Mosby, 1998.
9. Cameron JL: Current Surgical Therapy, 6th ed. St. Louis: CV Mosby, 1998.
10. Robbins SL: Pathologic Basis of Disease, 5th ed. Philadelphia: WB Saunders, 1994.

11. Schwartz SI, Shires GT, Spencer FC. Principles of Surgery, 7th ed. New York: McGraw-Hill, 1999.
12. Brenner BM: The Kidney, 6th ed. Philadelphia: WB Saunders, 2000.
13. Fawcett D: A Textbook of Histology, 12th ed. New York: Chapman and Hall, 1994, p 404.
14. Fauci AS: Harrinson's Principles of Internal Medicine, 14th ed. New York: McGraw-Hill, 1998.
15. Gines P: Hepatorenal syndrome. Clin Liver Dis 4:487–507, 2000.
16. Feldman M, Scharschmidt BF, Sleisenger MG: Sleisenger and Fordtran's Gastrointestinal and Liver Disease, 6th ed. Philadelphia: WB Saunders, 1998.
17. Skandalakis JE, Skandalakis PN, Skandalakis LJ: Surgical Anatomy and Technique: A Pocket Manual, 2nd ed. New York: Springer, 1999.
18. O'Leary JP: The Physiologic Basis of Surgery, 2nd ed. Baltimore: Williams & Wilkins, 1996.
19. Gilman AG, Rall TW, Nies AS, Taylor P. The Pharmacologic Basis of Therapeutics, 8th ed. New York: Pergamon Press, 1990.
20. Wilson JD, Foster DW, Kronenberg HM, Larsen PR: Williams Textbook of Endocrinology, 9th ed. Philadelphia: WB Saunders, 1998.

NOTES

Fluids, Nutrition, and Electrolytes

QUESTIONS

1. The primary source of glucose for the cells in a patient in early starvation (1 week) comes from:
   a. Proteins in skeletal muscle
   b. Ketone bodies
   c. Free fatty acids
   d. Glycogenolysis
   e. Lipolysis and acetyl CoA
2. A 75-year-old woman underwent a Whipple procedure for pancreatic cancer. Her postoperative course was complicated with a stroke and an anastomotic leak requiring reexploration. She was still on mechanical ventilation on postoperative day 26, with two failed attempts at extubation. One reason that could explain this is a respiratory quotient of:
   a. 0.66
   b. 0.7
   c. 0.8
   d. 0.9
   e. 1.1
3. The energy requirements of a 70-kg resting man are approximately (kcal/day):
   a. 1400 to 1500
   b. 1600 to 1700
   c. 1800 to 1900
   d. 2000 to 2100
   e. 2200

4. Furosemide produces:
   a. Hypokalemia, hypocalciuria, hyponatremia, hypochlorhydria
   b. Generation of concentrated urine, hypocalciuria, hypokalemia
   c. Hypokalemia, hypocalcemia, increase in the driving force of water reabsorption
   d. Permanent deafness, hypokalemia, venodilation
   e. Hypokalemia, hyponatremia, hypocalcemia, hypochloremia

5. All of the following structures use glucose as primary fuel, except:
   a. Renal medulla
   b. Brain tissue
   c. White blood cells
   d. Peripheral nerves
   e. Heart

6. The principal metabolic fuel for colonocytes is:
   a. Butyrate
   b. Acetoacetate
   c. D-Glucose
   d. Glutamine
   e Propionate

7. Which of the following blood products has the lowest transfusion-associated risk of hepatitis C virus transmission?
   a. Apheresis platelets
   b. Irradiated packed red blood cells
   c. Washed red blood cells
   d. Albumin
   e. Cryoprecipitate

8. A 75-year-old black man comes to the emergency room with a history of lower gastrointestinal bleeding for 2 days. He is thirsty and cold.

On physical examination, he seems agitated and his skin is cold to touch. He is tachycardic and has postural hypotension. What is the circulating blood volume loss of this patient?
a. 10% to 20%
b. 20% to 30%
c. 30% to 40%
d. 40% to 50%
e. >50%

9. A 24-year-old man came into the emergency room after being involved in a house fire. You notice that he has carbonaceous sputum and that 65% of his full-thickness total body surface area is burned. Subsequently, the patient is intubated without any difficulty. End-tidal carbon dioxide is positive, and bilateral breath sounds are present. He suddenly experiences electrocardiographic changes and goes into cardiac arrest. Which of the following drugs is most likely responsible for this event?
   a. Etomidate
   b. Rocuronium
   c. Succinylcholine
   d. Midazolam
   e. Ketamine

10. What is the most common transfusion reaction?
    a. Fever
    b. Abdominal pain
    c. Rash
    d. Pruritus
    e. Jaundice

11. Which one of the following findings is most common in patients with primary hyperaldosteronism?
    a. Hypotension
    b. Hyperkalemia

c. Glucose intolerance
d. Hyper-reninism
e. Edema

12. What is the total body water deficit in a 70-kg male patient with a plasma sodium of 160 mEq/L?
    a. 2.5 L
    b. 3.5 L
    c. 4.5 L
    d. 5.5 L
    e. 6.5 L

13. Which associated electrolyte abnormality can cause a state of hypokalemia refractory to potassium replacement?
    a. Hypocalcemia
    b. Hypomagnesemia
    c. Hypophosphatemia
    d. Hypercalcemia
    e. Hyperphosphatemia

14. Which one of the following is *not* associated with hypomagnesemia?
    a. Torsades de pointes
    b. Ataxia
    c. Metabolic acidosis
    d. Diffuse muscle spasms
    e. Hyporeflexia

15. What is the most common cause of hypophosphatemia in the hospitalized patient?
    a. Use of enemas and antacids
    b. Diabetic ketoacidosis
    c. Respiratory alkalosis
    d. Sepsis
    e. Glucose loading

16. Which of the following is *not* a cause of metabolic acidosis with an increased anion gap?

a. Renal failure
b. Methanol intoxication
c. Diarrhea
d. Ketoacidosis
e. Lactic acidosis

17. What is the most prevalent anion of the intracellular fluid?
    a. Bicarbonate
    b. Chloride
    c. Phosphate
    d. Proteins
    e. Organic ions

18. What is the plasma osmolality of a patient with the following electrolyte profile:

Na^+: 145 mEq/L	Albumin: 3.0 g/dL
K^+: 5.0 mEq/L	Bilirubin: 1.5
Cl^-: 110 mEq/L	Ca^{2+}: 8.5 mEq/L
HCO_3^-: 29 mEq/L	Mg^{2+}: 2.5 mEq/L
BUN: 28 mg/dL	Phosphate: 3.5 mEq/L
Creatinine: 1.0 mg/dL	Glucose: 180 mg/dL

    a. 275
    b. 297
    c. 305
    d. 310
    e. 320

19. Regarding perioperative management of the diabetic patient, which one of the following statements is incorrect?
    a. Oral hypoglycemic agents should be discontinued 24 hours before surgery.
    b. Intermediate- and long-lasting insulin should be discontinued on the morning of the operation.
    c. Blood glucose levels should be monitored every 30 minutes, until stable at 150 to

200 mg/100 mL, then hourly until the patient is awake.

d. The treatment of severe hyperglycemia must precede any surgical intervention.
e. The most common perioperative complications of patients with diabetes are related to hypoglycemia.

ANSWERS

1. METABOLIC EFFECTS OF STARVATION: correct answer a

During starvation, the hormone insulin decreases and the metabolic processes are directed to mobilize fat, carbohydrate, and protein. In early starvation, the glycogen reserves are depleted quickly (48 to 72 hours of fasting). Body fat, however, contains large energy stores in most patients. It would be ideal if all of the energy needs in starvation could be met from stored carbohydrate and fat, but studies have shown that in starvation this is not the case. Once the liver glycogen reserves are exhausted, the body adjusts by hydrolyzing skeletal muscle proteins and using the amino acids as sources of glucose. During 7 days of starvation, as much as 500 g of protein, or 5% of the total body intracellular protein, may be lost. The metabolic response to starvation may continue for extended periods, with little health risk, until approximately 20% to 30% of the initial starting weight is lost.[1]

In prolonged starvation, adaptive mechanisms conserve protein by enabling a greater portion of the energy needs to be met by fat metabolism, with a decreased requirement for glucose. The production of ketone bodies from fatty acid is accelerated, and the brain gets a significant proportion of its energy from these ketones. The principal energy substrate is adipose tissue (60%).[2]

2. RESPIRATORY QUOTIENT: correct answer e

The respiratory quotient (RQ) is defined as the ratio of the volume of carbon dioxide produced to the volume of oxygen used on oxidation of a given nutrient. The value for carbohydrate is very close to 1.0, whereas that for fat is around 0.7, for protein 0.81, and for alcohol 0.66. The RQ is a useful guide to the mixture of nutrients being oxidized, and if the protein oxidation can be determined from urinary nitrogen and there is little alcohol in the diet, the amounts of fat and carbohydrate oxidized can be calculated. Over 24 hours, the RQ should reflect the diet composition if the patient is in energy balance. On a normal Western diet of 35% energy as fat and 15% energy as protein, the 24-hour RQ should be around 0.87.[3]

Respiratory failure requiring ventilatory assistance or difficulty in weaning patients from respirators may occur if excess glucose is provided. In this case, the RQ may rise rapidly to values >1.[4]

3. ENERGY REQUIREMENTS: correct answer a

The average resting postabsorptive 70-kg man consumes oxygen at a rate of about 200 mL/min, or 288 L/day. This equals about 1450 kcal/day. In general, energy needs increase as illness severity increases: uncomplicated postoperative (1500 to 1700 kcal/day), sepsis (2000 to 2400 kcal/day), multiple trauma and mechanical ventilation (2200 to 2600 kcal/day), and major burn (2500 to 3000 kcal/day).[5]

4. LOOP DIURETICS: correct answer e

Loop diuretics (furosemide, bumetanide, ethacrynic acid, torsemide) inhibit the Na^+,K^+ $2Cl^-$ reabsorptive pump at the thick ascending limb of the loop of Henle, causing a diuresis of NaCl and KCl. At this nephron site, 20% to 30% of filtered sodium is reabsorbed. Since loop diuretics can cause excretion of about 20% of filtered sodium, it is apparent that these agents can block virtually all reabsorption by this segment of the nephron. In doing so, the segment becomes metabolically quiescent, accounting for the protective effect of loop diuretics against ischemic insults. The loop of Henle normally borders on hypoxemia: metabolic oxygen demands are great, whereas oxygen saturation is relatively low in this region of the kidney. Thus, the loop is uniquely susceptible to ischemic insults. By minimizing oxygen demands, loop diuretics can be protective. Since a major component of calcium reabsorption occurs parallel to that of sodium at the thick ascending limb, loop diuretics enhance calcium excretion sufficiently to be a useful therapeutic adjunct in patients with hypercalcemia. However, their use should be reserved until the volume depletion associated with hypercalcemia is corrected with infusions of saline.[6]

Loop diuretics also have a short-lasting venodilating effect when administered intravenously. This explains the immediate improvement that often occurs in patients with acute pulmonary edema, before any diuresis has occurred. The venodilation results in decreased cardiac preload, a fall in pulmonary artery wedge pressure, and symptomatic relief.

The most commonly encountered adverse effects of loop diuretics are intravascular volume depletion and hypokalemia. Chronic use usually leads to hypochloremic metabolic alkalosis. In addition, they can cause both auditory and vestibular toxicity. Although deafness is usually transient when caused by furosemide, there are reports of permanent hearing loss following ethacrynic acid administration.[7]

5. BODY ENERGY STORES: correct answer e

Because several vital organs, including the brain, peripheral nerves, renal medulla, red blood cells, white blood cells, and inflammatory tissue, all use glucose as primary fuel, the need for an ongoing glucose supply is imperative if the organism is to survive. An ongoing glucose supply is provided via proteolysis (primarily skeletal muscle) and accelerated hepatic gluconeogenesis. The conversion of amino acids to glucose is a necessary step because the enzymatic machinery is not present in humans to convert long-chain fatty acids to glucose.[8]

6. SHORT-CHAIN FATTY ACIDS: correct answer a

Acetoacetate, propionate, and butyrate are produced by fermentation of soluble pectin by colonic bacteria. Only 10% of acetoacetate is used locally, with 90% exported into the portal vein. With propionate, 50% is exported; with β-hydroxybutyrate, 80% is consumed locally by the colonocyte and only 20% enters the portal vein. Compared with other common fuels, butyrate is the principal metabolic fuel for colonocytes, with acetoacetate, L-glutamine, and D-glucose following in sequential order of importance. Butyrate stimulates ketogenesis, adenosine triphosphate generation, lipolysis, and absorption of sodium and potassium. Because short-chain fatty acids are not synthesized endogenously, the colonic mucosa can only obtain these respiratory fuels from bacterial fermentation.[9]

7. TRANSFUSION: correct answer d

Human albumin is a product derived from blood collected from volunteer donors. In addition to sterilization by filtration, albumin is heated for 10 hours at 60°C. This procedure has been shown to be effective in inactivating hepatitis virus. Albumin is a highly soluble protein, accounting for 80% of the colloid osmotic pressure of the plasma. Albumin has been used for the treatment of hypovolemia, burns, and cirrhosis as well as during coronary bypass surgery. Adverse reactions to albumin are extremely rare, although nausea, fever, chills, or urticaria may occur.

Apheresis is an effective way to harvest platelets from a single donor. One unit of platelet pheresis may replace 4 to 8 units of regular platelets. Usually, platelets collected by apheresis contain few leukocytes. If the leukocyte content is less than 5×10^6 and the platelet count is more than 3×10^{11}, the unit can be considered leukocyte-reduced. Pheresis does not reduce the risk of hepatitis C virus (HCV) infection.

Lymphocytes contained in blood products can be irradiated to prevent their proliferation, which can cause graft-versus-host disease. Blood products are exposed to a source of gamma irradiation, receiving a dose around 2500 cGy. Irradiation does not prevent the transmission of HCV.[10]

Washed components of blood are prepared by washing blood cells with 0.9% sodium chloride, with or without small amounts of dextran. Washed blood is indicated (1) if plasma contains antibodies known to be harmful for the intended recipient or (2) to remove constituents to which the intended recipient is known to have side effects, that is, removal of antibodies such as anti-IgA. Washed blood products and unwashed blood products carry the same risk of HCV transmission.

Cryoprecipitate is prepared by thawing fresh-frozen plasma between 1°C and 6°C and recovering the precipitate. Cryoprecipitate provides factor VIII, fibrinogen, von Willebrand factor, and factor XIII and is considered a second-line agent in the treatment of von Willebrand disease and hemophilia A. Cryoprecipitate is also used to control bleeding associated with fibrinogen deficiency and to treat factor XIII deficiency. Cryoprecipitate has the same risk of other blood products regarding HCV transmission.[11]

8. BLOOD LOSS: correct answer c

The signs and symptoms of hypovolemic or hemorrhagic shock depend on the degree of the intravascular depletion, duration, and compensatory reactions to hypovolemia. Blood flow is progressively reduced to skin, kidneys and viscera, heart, and ultimately brain. The clinical findings correlate with the blood volume redistribution and involved organs.

The response to a blood loss of less than 15% is vasoconstriction, and clinical findings may be absent.

Patients who have lost less than 20% of their blood volume present with pale and cool skin, tachycardia, and normal blood pressure.

When a patient has lost 20% to 40% of the circulating blood volume, oliguria, postural hypotension, and restlessness ensue.

When more than 40% of blood volume is lost, altered mental status is present, varying from agitation to unresponsiveness, along with the previous signs and symptoms described plus hypotension.[12, 13]

9. HYPERKALEMIA: correct answer c

Succinylcholine is a depolarizing skeletal muscle relaxant. It combines with acetylcholine receptors of the postsynaptic motor plate to cause depolarization. The first phase of the neuromuscular blockade consists of fasciculations followed by complete muscle relaxation with paralysis, occurring in less than 1 minute after intravenous administration of the drug. The usual dose is 1 to 2 mg/kg and lasts approximately 4 to 6 minutes.[14]

Succinylcholine is hydrolyzed by plasma cholinesterase, and 10% of the drug is excreted unchanged in the urine. No hepatic or renal metabolism occurs. Succinylcholine is contraindicated in patients with major burns, multiple trauma, or extensive denervation of skeletal muscle because of the risk of hyperkalemia, which may result in cardiac arrest.

Succinylcholine is also contraindicated in patients with a family history of malignant hyperthermia, skeletal muscle myopathies, and known hypersensitivity to the drug.

Malignant hyperthermia presents usually with increased carbon dioxide expired production, muscle spasms that progress to rigidity, tachycardia, tachypnea, and hyperthermia. Treatment consists of discontinuing the anesthetics, correcting the acidosis, supporting circulation with optimization of the fluid status, and controlling body temperature. Dantrolene also should be used in the treatment of malignant hyperthermia.

Other side effects of succinylcholine include bradycardia, tachycardia, prolonged respiratory depression, increased intraocular pressure, jaw rigidity, and rhabdomyolysis leading to acute renal failure.[12, 15]

10. TRANSFUSION REACTIONS: correct answer a

Several undesirable transfusion reactions can occur, including hemolytic reaction, allergic reac-tion, non-hemolytic febrile reaction, cytopenic reactions, and tissue-organoimmunologic reactions. The most common reaction to blood transfusion is fever. This occurs just after the transfusion and is due to patient antibodies against donor leukocytes (leukoagglutinins); fever is considered a nonhemolytic reaction. In the past, these febrile episodes were attributed to a pyrogen contami-nation of the blood. Pyrogen contamination still occurs at a rate of approximately 2%. Aside from the fever, chills, malaise, headache, tachycardia, and even pulmonary infiltrates are possible. Symptoms are self-limited and disappear in 24 to 48 hours. The chance of having such transfusion reactions can be reduced using frozen packed red blood cells, washed packed red blood cells, or packed red blood cells previously filtered to reduce the leukocyte number. The second most common reaction to blood transfusion is an allergic reaction. Symptoms are localized or generalized hives, sometimes associated with asthma-like symptoms: bronchospasm, dyspnea, and stridor due to laryngeal edema. The response to antihistamines and epinephrine is excellent in these cases.

The following approach should be taken if the patient experiences a transfusion reaction:

1. Stop the blood transfusion.
2. Check vital signs. If the patient is hypotensive, start intravenous (IV) infusion of fluids and consider a dopamine drip at 5 μg/kg/min.
3. When the patient is stable, send blood for a Coomb test and a urine dipstick test for blood.[13, 16, 17]

11. PRIMARY HYPERALDOSTERONISM: correct answer c

The most common causes of primary hyperal dosteronism (PH) are adrenal adenoma (65%), idiopathic hyperaldosteronism (30%), and glucocorticoid-remediable aldosteronism (3%). Other uncommon causes of PH are adrenal carcinoma, congenital adrenal hyperplasia, licorice ingestion, and Liddle syndrome.

Patients usually present with fatigue and cramps due to the hypokalemic state, associated with hypertension and polyuria. The mineralocorticoid effect of sodium is lost on patients with PH, and edema is rarely seen clinically. High levels of aldosterone also suppress the secretion of renin, leading to a chronic state of hyporeninemia. Because of intracellular depletion of potassium, insulin secretion is impaired in many patients with PH, and glucose intolerance or diabetes may be present at the time of diagnosis.[12, 18]

12. FLUIDS AND ELECTROLYTES: correct answer c

The normal total body water (TBW) is usually 60% of the lean body weight (kg) in men and 50% in women. However, in hypernatremia, the normal TBW should be approximately 10% less than usual (50% in men and 40% in women). The product of TBW and plasma sodium should be a constant[13]:

Current TBW × Current plasma Na
= Normal TBW × Normal plasma Na

Current TBW × 160 = (0.5 × 70) × 140 (using 140 mEq/L as the normal plasma concentration of sodium)

Current TBW = 35 × 140/160

Current TBW = 4.5 L

TBW deficit = Normal TBW − Current TBW

TBW deficit = 35 − 30.5

TBW deficit = 4.5 L

13. FLUIDS AND ELECTROLYTES: correct answer b

Magnesium depletion impairs potassium reabsorption across the renal tubules. Magnesium repletion should be performed to achieve normal serum potassium levels.

Conversely, hypophosphatemia can lead to an increased magnesium excretion, causing hypomagnesemia. In these cases, hypophosphatemia should be corrected to ensure adequate levels of magnesium stores.[13]

14. FLUIDS AND ELECTROLYTES: correct answer e

Hypermagnesemia is associated mainly with delay of cardiac conduction and occurs in patients with renal insufficiency.

Hypomagnesemia occurs in several different conditions, including diabetes mellitus, acute myocardial infarction, diarrhea, and alcohol abuse. Hypomagnesemia is also associated with the use of furosemide, aminoglycosides, amphotericin, digitalis, cisplatin, total parenteral nutrition, cyclosporine, and nasogastric tube suctioning.

Signs and symptoms are cardiac arrhythmias, including torsade de pointes, ataxia, metabolic acidosis, slurred speech, diffuse muscle spasms, excessive salivation, seizures, hyperreflexia, and progressive obtundation.[13]

15. FLUIDS AND ELECTROLYTES: correct answer e

The most common cause of hypophosphatemia in the hospitalized patient is glucose loading, usually during refeeding alcoholic, malnourished, or debilitated patients.

The movement of glucose into the cells is accompanied by similar movement of phosphate, resulting in hypophosphatemia. A similar mechanism is responsible for hypophosphatemia in patients with respiratory alkalosis.

Sepsis may cause hypophosphatemia, probably through the increase of catecholamines, which also leads to a shift of phosphate into the cells. Osmotic diuresis and glycosuria cause excretion of extra amounts of phosphate in the urine, leading to hypophosphatemia.

Aluminum and other phosphorus-binding agents can form insoluble complexes with inor-ganic phosphorus, which prevents the absorption of phosphorus by the gastrointestinal tract, resulting in hypophosphatemia.[13]

16. FLUIDS AND ELECTROLYTES: correct answer c

Diarrhea is a cause of normal anion gap metabolic acidosis. The causes of metabolic acidosis can be divided into two different categories: with an increased anion gap and with normal anion gap. The anion gap, which has a normal value of 12 ± 4 mEq/L, represents the concentrations of anions that are present in the serum but are not routinely determined, such as phosphates and sulfates. The anion gap can be calculated by the following formula:

$$AG = (Na + K) - (Cl + HCO_3)$$

An increase in the anion gap represents an increase of one of those unmeasured acids. No change in the anion gap, with decrease in plasma bicarbonate and serum pH, suggests loss of bicarbonate.

Common causes of metabolic acidosis with increase anion gap are:

Renal failure
Lactic acidosis
Ketoacidosis
Intoxication with salicylates, ethylene glycol, and methanol

Common causes of metabolic acidosis with normal anion gap are:

Diarrhea
Pancreatic fistulas
Ureterosigmoidostomy
Renal tubular acidosis
Carbonic anhydrase inhibition[12, 19]

17. FLUIDS AND ELECTROLYTES: correct answer c

Phosphate is the most prevalent anion of the intracellular fluid. Proteins, sulfate, bicarbonate, and chloride are other common anions present in the intracellular space.

In the extracellular space, the most prevalent anion is chloride, followed by bicarbonate, proteins, organic acids, phosphate, and sulfate.[12, 19]

18. FLUIDS AND ELECTROLYTES: correct answer d

The concentration of the plasma osmolality can be calculated using the following formula:[13]

Plasma osmolality = 2 × Na + glucose/18 + BUN/2.8

$$= 2 \times 145 + 180/18 + 28/2.8$$

$$= 310 \text{ mOsm/ kg } H_2O$$

19. FLUIDS AND ELECTROLYTES: correct answer e

Fluid and electrolyte abnormalities, hypertension, and poor wound healing are the major risks in the hyperglycemic surgical patient, which are more common than the risks of hypoglycemia during insulin treatment in a well-monitored surgical patient.

Oral hypoglycemic agents should be discontinued 24 hours before surgery. Also, intermediate- or long-acting insulin should be held on the morning of the surgery. In some patients, infusion of glucose (D5W + 20 KCl/L at 100 mL/hour) together with an insulin infusion (25 units of insulin on 250 mL normal saline at 1 to 2 units/hour) should be considered. Blood glucose should be monitored every 30 minutes until stable at 150 to 200 mg/100 mL, then hourly until the patient is awake, and every hour until the diet is resumed.

The treatment of severe hyperglycemia must precede any surgical intervention and should be accomplished as soon as possible, avoiding delay of the surgical procedure.[12]

Quick Answers

1. A	6. A	11. C	16. C
2. E	7. D	12. C	17. C
3. A	8. C	13. B	18. D
4. E	9. C	14. E	19. E
5. E	10. A	15. E	

REFERENCES

1. Zeman F: Clinical Nutrition and Dietetics, 2nd ed. New York: Macmillan, 1991, pp 554–556.
2. Zaloga G: Nutrition in Critical Care, 1st ed. St. Louis: CV Mosby, 1994, pp 12–13.
3. Garrow JS: Human Nutrition and Dietetics, 10th ed. New York: Churchill Livingstone, 2000, pp 28–29.
4. Zeman F: Clinical Nutrition and Dietetics, 2nd ed. New York: Macmillan, 1991, p 142.
5. Greenfield L: Surgery: Scientific Principles and Practice, 2nd ed. Philadelphia: Lippincott, 1997, pp 44–45.
6. Munson P: Principles of Pharmacology, 1st ed. New York: Chapman and Hall, 1995, pp 664–666.
7. Kalant H, Roschlau W: Principles of Medical Pharmacology, 6th ed. New York: Oxford University Press, 1998, pp 516–517.
8. Sabiston D: The Biological Basis of Modern Surgical Practice, 15th ed. Philadelphia: WB Saunders, 1997, pp 57–58.
9. Sabiston D: The Biological Basis of Modern Surgical Practice, 15th ed. Philadelphia: WB Saunders, 1997, p 149.
10. Schreiber GB, Busch MP, Kleinman SH, et al: The risk of transfusion-transmitted viral infections. N Engl J Med 334:1685–1690, 1996.
11. Gerety RJ, Aronson DL: Plasma derivants and viral hepatitis. Transfusion 22:347–351, 1982.
12. Townsend CM, Beauchamp RD, Evers BM, Mattox K: Sabiston Textbook of Surgery, 16th ed. Philadelphia: WB Saunders, 2001.
13. Marino PL: The ICU Book, 2nd ed. Baltimore: Williams & Wilkins, 1998.
14. Miller RD: Anesthesia, 5th ed. Philadelphia: Churchill Livingstone, 2000.
15. Rosen P: Emergency Medicine: Concepts and Clinical Practice, 4th ed. St. Louis: CV Mosby, 1998.

16. King KE: Treating anemia. Hematol Oncol Clin North Am 10:1305–1320, 1996.
17. Cotran RS, Kumar V, Collins C: Robbins Pathologic Basis of Disease, 6th ed. Philadelphia: WB Saunders, 1999.
18. Wilson JD: Williams Textbook of Endocrinology, 9th ed. Philadelphia: WB Saunders, 1998.
19. Brenner BM: The Kidney, 6th ed. Philadelphia: WB Saunders, 2000.

NOTES

Hemostasis and Wound Healing

QUESTIONS

1. Regarding the factor V Leiden mutation, which of the following statements is false?
   a. It is the most common inheritable thrombophilia.
   b. It results in resistance to activated protein C.
   c. It causes a fivefold higher incidence of deep venous thrombosis.
   d. At least 90% of patients with the mutation exhibit a clinical propensity for thrombosis even in the absence of other risk factors for thrombosis (history of deep venous thrombosis, pulmonary embolism [PE], obesity).
   e. Patients with the mutation undergoing a major surgical procedure should be treated prophylactically with low-molecular-weight heparin (LMWH).
2. Regarding wound healing, which of the following statements is false?
   a. Dermal appendages such as sweat glands and hair follicles can repair themselves in a partial-thickness injury but cannot regenerate in full-thickness wounds.
   b. Type III collagen is initially more predominant in wounds than in normal skin, but as the wound matures, type I collagen is deposited in increasing amounts, and by the time wound healing is completed, it is the predominant collagen.

c. Transforming growth factor β is released from platelets, fibroblasts, and macrophages in the wound and stimulates the deposition of collagen, enhances angiogenesis, and is chemotactic for fibroblasts, monocytes, and macrophages.
d. Hypoxia causes accumulation of lactate in the cell, which can stimulate collagen synthesis by increasing collagen gene transcription and increased prolyl hydroxylase activity.
e. Tenascin is a matrix glycoprotein that enhances the cell adhesion effects of fibronectin.

3. All of the following statements concerning drugs that affect hemostasis are true except:
   a. Coumadin is contraindicated during lactation.
   b. Heparin induces a conformational change in anti-thrombin III, inhibiting factors IIa and Xa.
   c. The protein C enzyme system downregulates coagulation by proteolytically inactivating the two essential protein cofactors of the cascade, factors V and VIII.
   d. Coumadin skin necrosis is more common in patients with hereditary deficiency of protein C.
   e. Ticlopidine is an inhibitor of platelet function. Platelets from patients taking this drug do not bind fibrinogen.

4. Compared with heparin, LMWH has the following characteristics, except:
   a. Like heparin, LMHW produces its major anticoagulant effect by activating antithrombin III.
   b. LMHW has reduced ability to catalyze inactivation of thrombin because the smaller fragments cannot bind to thrombin, but they retain their ability to inactivate factor Xa.

   c. Nonspecific binding to plasma proteins is reduced, with a corresponding improvement in the predictability of their dose-response relationship.
   d. LMHW has reduced binding to macrophages and endothelial cells, with an associated increase in plasma half-life.
   e. LMWH is cleared principally by the hepatic route.

5. All of the following are true regarding heparin and heparin-induced thrombocytopenia, except:
   a. LMWH is contraindicated for the treatment of heparin-induced thrombocytopenia.
   b. Heparin produces a conformational change in antithrombin III and therefore markedly accelerates its ability to inactivate the coagulation enzymes thrombin (factor IIa), factor Xa, and factor IXa.
   c. Heparin is not absorbed after oral administration and therefore must be given by injection.
   d. The timing of thrombocytopenia, in the immune form of heparin-induced thrombocytopenia, is influenced by the presence or absence of prior exposure to heparin.
   e. Arterial thrombosis is more common than venous thrombosis (ratio, approximately 4:1) in patients with heparin-induced thrombocytopenia.

6. All of the following are true about adverse effects of oral anticoagulant therapy, except:
   a. The risk of major bleeding has been reported to be increased by age >65 years.
   b. Atrial fibrillation increases the risk of major bleeding.

c. An association has been reported between warfarin-induced skin necrosis and protein C deficiency and, less commonly, protein S deficiency, but this complication can also occur in nondeficient persons.
d. Oral anticoagulants cross the placenta and can produce a characteristic embryopathy, central nervous system abnormalities, or fetal bleeding.
e. There is convincing evidence that warfarin does induce an anticoagulant effect in the breast-fed infant when the drug is administered to a nursing mother.

7. Indications for placement of an inferior vena cava filter include all of the following, except:
   a. Contraindication to anticoagulation after an episode of iliofemoral vein thrombosis
   b. Documented previous episode of pulmonary embolism with no other risk factors
   c. High-risk condition for fatal pulmonary embolism
   d. No history of vein thrombosis but long-term prophylaxis is necessary (paraplegic patient)
   e. Free-floating thrombus

8. What is the most common major adverse reaction to protamine sulfate when it is given for the reversal of heparin anticoagulation?
   a. Severe hypotension
   b. Acute pulmonary vasoconstriction
   c. Anaphylactic shock
   d. Acute pulmonary bronchoconstriction
   e. Pulmonary embolism

9. After wound healing has occurred, the tensile strength of the scar compared with normal skin is:
   a. 60% to 70%

b. 70% to 80%
c. 80% to 90%
d. 90% to 100%
e. 100%

10. The rate-limiting factor in wound healing is:
    a. Oxygen
    b. Cyclic adenosine monophosphate
    c. Collagen synthesis
    d. Angiogenesis
    e. Polymorphonuclear cell function

11. What is responsible for the production of von Willebrand factor?
    a. Macrophages
    b. Neutrophils
    c. Endothelial cells
    d. Platelets
    e. Fibroblasts

12. Regarding wound healing, what is the correct sequence of cell appearance in the wound?
    a. Platelets, neutrophils, macrophages, fibroblasts
    b. Neutrophils, macrophages, platelets, fibroblasts
    c. Macrophages, neutrophils, fibroblasts, platelets
    d. Platelets, macrophages, neutrophils, fibroblasts
    e. Fibroblasts, neutrophils, macrophages, platelets

13. A 25-year-old African American woman develops a large keloid at her appendectomy incision site. The predominant collagen found in this lesion is most likely:
    a. Type I
    b. Type II

c. Type III
d. Type IV
e. Type IX

ANSWERS

1. FACTOR V LEIDEN (FVL) MUTATION: correct answer d

The most common inheritable thrombophilia is the FVL mutation, which results in resistance to activated protein C with the potential for causing spontaneous intravascular clotting. This is manifested primarily as spontaneous venous thrombosis but can occasionally cause pulmonary embolus and, less commonly, arterial obstruction. It is estimated that 5% to 6% of white subjects are heterozygous for FVL mutation and are potentially hypercoagulable. FVL mutation causes a fivefold higher incidence of deep venous thrombosis than occurs in the normal patient, but the incidence of pulmonary embolism is half the anticipated frequency in those patients. Many patients (at least 90%) do not exhibit a clinical propensity for thrombosis unless the genetic mutation is accompanied by one of several risk factors, including previous history of spontaneous venous thrombosis, previous pulmonary emboli, or spontaneous arterial thrombosis, especially coronary or cerebral vascular occlusion in patients younger than age 50 without a prominent smoking history. Routine testing is uniformly considered to be cost-prohibitive in preoperative patients without significant risk factors; studies done in this population have shown that screening for this mutation does not appear to offer additional benefit in terms of preventing postoperative death from acute pulmonary embolism. However, in patients who are prescribed tamoxifen, it is important to obtain the same history and to assess risk factors as though the patient were a surgical candidate. With a positive history, FVL assays should be obtained.

In preoperative patients with the FVL mutation, the best anticoagulant prophylaxis available is LMWH (enoxaparin, 40 to 60 mg daily, subcutaneously) unless there is a significant contraindication or the operation will be of short duration, requiring less than 1 hour of general anesthesia.[1–4]

2. WOUND HEALING: correct answer e

Tenascin is a matrix glycoprotein that inhibits the cell adhesion effect of fibronectin and permits cells to detach from the matrix and migrate. The appearance of tenascin in the wound matrix correlates with the initiation of epithelial and mesenchymal cell migration.

The control mechanisms for collagen synthesis involves several steps: Lactate and hypoxia reduce the nicotinamide adenine dinucleotide (NAD^+) pool by converting NAD^+ to NADH. This reduces the amount of the metabolite of NAD^+, adenosine diphosphoribose (ADPR). The polymerized form of ADPR also normally downregulates collagen gene transcription in the resting state. Prolyl hydroxylase is also inhibited by ADPR.

The sustained production of tumor growth factor β (TGF-β) at the wound site leads to tissue fibrosis. Platelets and macrophages release TGF-β at the injury site. To repair the damage, TGF-β induces the deposition of extracellular matrix by simultaneously stimulating the production of new matrix protein (fibronectin, collagens, and proteoglycans), blocking matrix degradation by decreasing the synthesis of proteases and increasing the synthesis of protease inhibitors, and modulating the expression of cell surface integrins in a manner that enhances cell-matrix interaction and matrix assembly. TGF-β also induces its own production by cells, thus amplifying its biologic effects.[5]

3. DRUGS AFFECTING HEMOSTASIS: correct answer a

The anticoagulant activity of heparin is the result of its high-affinity interaction with antithrombin III. This induces a conformational change in antithrombin III and confers activity on the complex as a potent inhibitor of coagulation factors IIa (thrombin) and Xa. LMWH preparations have a greater anti-Xa activity per unit of anti-IIa activity than do standard heparins. The plasma half-lives of LMWH preparations are approximately twice that of standard heparins.

When activated, the protein C (PC) enzyme system downregulates coagulation by proteolytically inactivating the two essential protein cofactors of the cascade, factors V and VIII. Activation of PC to PCa occurs by the proteolytic action of thrombin. Circulating thrombin, however, does not activate PC; rather, thrombin binds to thrombomodulin, a protein on the surface of vascular endothelial cells, changing its specificity so that it no longer cleaves fibrinogen but instead activates PC. PCa, in conjunction with a cofactor on cell surfaces, protein S, then inactivates factors V and VIII.

Most proteins of the coagulation system are synthesized in the liver. Factors II, VII, IX, and X and proteins C and S contain an unusual modified amino acid, gamma-carboxylated glutamic acid. This post-translational modification is accomplished by a vitamin K-dependent carboxylase. Oral anticoagulants work by inhibiting vitamin K. An unusual complication of these drugs is skin necrosis, due to thrombotic occlusion of small dermal vessels, usually in the extremities, buttocks, abdominal wall, or breasts. This usually occurs early in the course of therapy and may be due to the transient generation of a "hypercoagulable" state induced by rapid falls in protein C levels prior to the decrease in factors II, VII, IX, and X. Patients with hereditary deficiency of protein C are at higher risk for this complication. The coumarins cross the placenta and are teratogenic in the 6th through 12th weeks of gestation. They are therefore contraindicated during the first half of pregnancy only. They do not appear in milk.

Ticlopidine is an inhibitor of platelet function. Platelets from patients taking this drug do not bind fibrinogen in response to most agonists, suggesting that they are incapable of generating a functional fibrinogen receptor.[6]

4. LOW-MOLECULAR-WEIGHT HEPARIN: correct answer e

Compared with heparin, LMWHs have the following characteristics: (1) reduced ability to catalyze inactivation of thrombin because the smaller fragments cannot bind to thrombin but retain their ability to inactivate factor Xa, (2) reduced nonspecific binding to plasma proteins, with a corresponding improvement in the predictability of their dose-response relationship, (3) reduced binding to macrophages and endothelial cells, with an associated increase in their plasma half-life, (4) reduced binding to platelets and PF4, which may explain the lower incidence of heparin-induced thrombocytopenia, and (5) possibly reduced binding to osteoblasts that results in less activation of osteoclasts and an associated reduction in bone loss. LMWHs are cleared principally by the renal route, and their biologic half-life is increased in patients with renal failure.

Like heparin, LMWHs produce their major anticoagulant effect by activating antithrombin. Also, they do not cross the placental barrier, and a descriptive study suggests that they may be safe and effective in pregnancy.[7]

5. HEPARIN-INDUCED THROMBOCYTOPENIA: correct answer e

Heparin is a glycosaminoglycan composed of chains of alternating residues of D-glucosamine and an uronic acid. Its major anticoagulant effect is accounted for by a unique pentasaccharide with a high-affinity binding sequence to antithrombin III (ATIII) that is present in only one third of heparin molecules. The anticoagulant effect of heparin is mediated largely through its interaction with ATIII; this produces a conformational change in ATIII and therefore markedly accelerates its ability to inactivate the coagulation enzymes thrombin (factor IIa), factor Xa, and factor IXa. Of these three enzymes, thrombin is the most sensitive to inhibition by heparin/ATIII. Heparin is not absorbed after oral administration and therefore must be given by injection. The two preferred routes of administration are IV and subcutaneous. Intramuscular (IM) injection can produce large hematomas caused by accidental puncture of an IM vein and therefore should be avoided. There is evidence that heparin administered by intermittent IV injection is associated with more bleeding than when it is administered by the continuous IV route; the latter method is therefore preferred if heparin is administered intravenously. The efficacy and safety of heparin administered by either the continuous IV method or the subcutaneous route are comparable provided that the dosages used are adequate.

Thrombocytopenia is a well-recognized complication of heparin therapy. Two forms of thrombocytopenia are described: an early benign, reversible nonimmune thrombocytopenia and a late, more serious IgG-mediated immune thrombocytopenia. The relationship of nonimmune heparin-associated thrombocytopenia with heparin use is uncertain since the platelet count recovers in these patients despite continued heparin treatment. In contrast, the immune form of heparin-induced thrombocytopenia (HIT) is characterized by strong IgG-mediated platelet activation and is associated with a substantial risk of thrombotic complications. The timing of thrombocytopenia is influenced by the presence or absence of prior exposure to heparin. The platelet count begins to fall 5 to 10 days after heparin therapy is started in a previously unexposed person with HIT, although overt thrombocytopenia may not be reached for a few more days. In contrast, thrombocytopenia may occur within 24 hours of exposure to heparin in patients who have been exposed previously to heparin; this rapid onset of thrombocytopenia generally occurs in patients who have received heparin within the previous 3 months, an observation that suggests that preexisting IgG, rather than an anamnestic response, is responsible for the rapid platelet count fall. Venous thrombosis is more common than arterial thrombosis (ratio, approximately 4:1) in patients with HIT.

A newly recognized syndrome, *venous limb gangrene,* is characterized by acral (distal) tissue losses associated with extensive venous thrombosis that involves both large veins and small venules. This disorder, which may explain more than half the limb loss attributable to HIT, has been linked to acquired deficiency of protein C during warfarin therapy of deep venous thrombosis complicating HIT. One of the anticoagulant drugs, danaparoid sodium, or the recombinant hirudin lepirudin, should be used to treat acute HIT complicated by thrombosis. Anticoagulation with one of these agents until the platelet count has recovered should also be considered in patients with acute HIT without thrombosis, as there is evidence for a high risk for thrombosis in these patients. Warfarin should not be used alone to treat acute HIT complicated by deep venous thrombosis because of the risk of causing venous limb gangrene. However, warfarin appears to be safe in acute HIT when it is given to a patient who is adequately anticoagulated with a drug that reduces thrombin generation in HIT, such as danaparoid sodium or lepirudin, although it is recommended that warfarin therapy be delayed until the platelet count has risen to above 100,000. LMWH is contraindicated for the treatment of acute HIT.[7]

6. ORAL ANTICOAGULANT SIDE EFFECTS: correct answer e

Bleeding is the main complication of oral anticoagulant therapy. The risk of bleeding is influenced by the intensity of anticoagulant therapy, by the patient's underlying clinical disorder, and by the concomitant use of aspirin, which both impairs platelet function and produces gastric erosions; when used in very high doses, aspirin impairs synthesis of vitamin K-dependent clotting factors. The risk of major bleeding has been reported to be increased by age 65 years, a history of stroke or gastrointestinal bleeding, atrial fibrillation, and the presence of serious comorbid conditions such as renal insufficiency or anemia.

The most important nonhemorrhagic side effect of warfarin is skin necrosis. This uncommon complication usually occurs on the third to eighth day of therapy and is caused by extensive thrombosis of the venules and capillaries within the subcutaneous fat. An association has been reported between warfarin-induced skin necrosis, protein C deficiency and, less commonly, protein S deficiency, but this complication can also occur in nondeficient persons. The pathogenesis of this striking complication is unknown. A role for protein C deficiency seems probable and is supported by the similarity of the lesions to those seen in neonatal purpura fulminans that complicates homozygous protein C deficiency. The reason for the unusual localization of the lesions remains a mystery. The treatment of patients with warfarin-induced skin necrosis who require life-long anticoagulant therapy is problematic. Warfarin is considered to be contraindicated, and long-term heparin therapy is inconvenient and associated with osteoporosis. A reasonable approach in such patients is to restart warfarin therapy at a low dose, for example, 2 mg, under the coverage of therapeutic doses of heparin and to increase the warfarin dosage gradually over several weeks. This approach should avoid an abrupt fall in protein C levels before the levels of factors II, IX, and X are reduced and has been shown to be free of recurrence of skin necrosis in a number of case reports.

Oral anticoagulants cross the placenta and can produce a characteristic embryopathy, central nervous system abnormalities, or fetal bleeding. Warfarin should not be used in the first trimester of pregnancy and, if possible, it should also be avoided throughout the entire pregnancy. In some cases, however, in which the risk of embolism is high and full-dose heparin cannot be used (e.g., a mechanical heart valve treated with warfarin) or in which a temporary loss of therapeutic control would be life-threatening, a decision to continue warfarin therapy throughout pregnancy can be justified. Heparin is preferred when anticoagulants are indicated in pregnancy. There is convincing evidence that warfarin does not induce an anticoagulant effect in the breast-fed infant when the drug is administered to a nursing mother.[8]

7. INFERIOR VENA CAVA FILTERS: correct answer b

The most common inferior vena cava (IVC) filter used is the Greenfield filter. It has a conical shape, which gives this filter a structural advantage in that 75% of the basket can be filled with thrombus, without any compromise of the flow of the vessel. The filters are placed percutaneously, most frequently through the femoral or internal jugular veins. The reported incidence of pulmonary embolism with a vena cava filter is 2% to 5%.

The indications for IVC filter are:

1. Documented iliofemoral vein thrombosis and:
   Contraindication to anticoagulation
   Documented pulmonary embolism during full anticoagulation
   Free-floating thrombus
   High-risk condition for a fatal pulmonary embolism such as severe pulmonary disease
2. No iliofemoral vein thrombosis, but:
   Need for long-term prophylaxis, as in paraplegics
   High risk of thromboembolism and hemorrhage

One single episode of pulmonary embolism, without any other risk factors, is not an indication for an IVC filter placement.[9]

8. PROTAMINE SIDE EFFECTS: correct answer a

Protamines are proteins found in fish sperm. Since their discovery, protamines have earned a major role in human pharmacotherapy, including use in retarding the absorption of insulin (i.e., neutral protamine Hagedorn) and for the reversal of heparin anticoagulation. Adverse responses to protamine sulfate have been identified for many years. The incidence of adverse reactions to protamine has been reported to vary from 0.06% to 10.7%. Hemodynamic changes in systemic or pulmonary vasculature, or both, are the most commonly reported unintended response to protamine. In a series of 27 patients with adverse reactions, 25 had hypotension.[10]

9. WOUND HEALING: correct answer c

The tensile strength of the scar is approximately 85% compared with the normal skin.[11]

10. WOUND HEALING: correct answer a

Oxygen is essential for maintaining cellular integrity, function, and repair when tissues are injured. Evidence suggests that oxygen is the rate-limiting step in wound healing. Larger wounds may have significantly increased metabolic demands and larger areas of compromised microvascular oxygen delivery, limiting the healing process. In a normal host, healing may be delayed but may eventually occur as progressive microcapillary neovascularization ensues and oxygen delivery is restored. Problems occur in the patient with either compromised oxygen delivery or enhanced oxygen utilization, in whom the oxygen supply never meets oxygen demand and a chronic wound situation develops.[12]

11. VON WILLEBRAND FACTOR (vWF): correct answer c

vWF is a heterogeneous plasma glycoprotein that is produced by endothelial cells. Its major function is to facilitate platelet adhesion to vascular subendothelium. Adhesion is made through the glycoprotein (Gp) Ib-IX platelet receptor. It also serves as a plasma carrier for factor VIII. The normal plasma level of vWF is 10 mg/L.[13]

Von Willebrand disease is one of the most common congenital bleeding disorders. There are three major types: Type I, the most common type, with a mild to moderate decrease in plasma vWF, is characterized by a normal prothrombin time, a mildly prolonged activated partial thromboplastin time (aPTT), abnormal bleeding time, and decreased levels of VIII:C and vWF:Ag. In type II, the functionality of vWF is decreased, which produces a decrease in the ristocetin cofactor assay (R:cof) (ristocetin assay measures the efficiency of vWF in agglutinate platelets in the presence of the antibiotic ristocetin).[14]

Near complete absence of factor VIII:C, wVF:Ag, and R:cof characterize von Willebrand disease type III. The patient presents with prolonged aPTT, abnormal bleeding time, and low platelet levels.

The administration of desmopressin acetate (DDAVP), 0.3 μg/kg, results in a normalization of the bleeding time and factor VIII and vWF activities. Cryoprecipitate is a second-line agent in the treatment of von Willebrand disease but is also effective in preventing and controlling bleeding.[15]

12. WOUND HEALING: correct answer a

The wound healing process can be divided into three phases: inflammation, proliferation, and maturation. Hemostasis is the first event after the skin is injured and is mainly due to platelet aggregation.

Subsequently, platelet aggregation leads to release of cytokines and growth factors, including platelet-derived growth factor and transforming growth factors α and β. Also, the breakdown of the complement cascade releases chemotactic agents, such as C5a, IL-8, and leukotriene B4, which results in a massive migration of inflammatory cells, especially neutrophils. After 48 hours, macrophages outnumber the neutrophils. Indeed, macrophages are essential for wound healing and can be considered the most important cell in the wound healing process. Macrophages phagocytize dead tissue and bacteria; secrete elastase, collagenase, and cytokines; and stimulate fibroblast proliferation and collagen production. Fibroblasts are mesenchymal cells present in the healing wound by the third day after the injury, marking the beginning of the proliferative phase. The proliferative phase is characterized by fibroblast multiplication and collagen deposition. By the third week after the injury, macrophages and fibroblasts disappear from the wound and collagen begins a long process of remodeling and maturation.

Important aspects of wound healing are:

Phase I—Inflammation, 0 to 72 hours (3 days): Hemostasis (platelet aggregation) is followed by migration of inflammatory cells. Epithelialization and angiogenesis also occur.

Phase II—Proliferation, 3 days to 3 weeks: Fibroblasts appear and collagen deposition begins. Wound contraction by myofibroblasts also occurs.

Phase III—Maturation, 3 weeks to 2 years: Collagen deposition is maximal at 21 days, but the tensile strength is approximately only 15%. The process of wound maturation increases the tensile strength and, by 6 weeks, it reaches 80% to 90% of its final strength. As the scar matures, type III collagen is replaced by type I collagen.[15, 16]

13. COLLAGEN TYPES: correct answer c

Keloid formation is an abnormal amount of collagen (predominantly type III) in the connective tissue, producing a large, bulging, tumorous scar. Keloids tend to occur in areas such as the face, neck, earlobes, sternum, and forearms. Keloids are more frequent in black female adolescents or young adults.

A hypertrophic scar is an overproduction of connective tissue (predominantly collagen type I), which flattens over the course of 1 to 2 years, whereas keloids persist and can extend beyond the site of injury.

Type I: High tensile strength; dermis 80%, scars, bone 90%, tendons
Type II: Structural protein, cartilage 50% (type IX as well), vitreous humor
Type III: Embryonic tissue, vessels, keloids, granulation tissue
Type IV: All basement membranes[16]

Quick Answers

1. D	5. E	9. C	13. C
2. E	6. E	10. A	
3. A	7. B	11. C	
4. E	8. A	12. A	

REFERENCES

1. Blaszyk H, Bjornsson J: Factor V Leiden and morbid obesity in fatal postoperative pulmonary embolism. Arch Surg 135:1410–1413, 2000.
2. Bounameaux H: Factor V Leiden paradox: risk of deep venous thrombosis but not pulmonary embolism. Lancet 356:182–183, 2000.

3. Bontempo FA: The factor V Leiden mutation: spectrum of thrombotic events and laboratory evaluation. J Vasc Surg 25:271–275, 1997.
4. Weitz IC: Tamoxifen-associated venous thrombosis and activated protein C resistance due to FVL. Cancer 79:2024–2027, 1997.
5. Sabiston D: The Biological Basis of Modern Surgical Practice, 15th ed. Philadelphia: WB Saunders, 1997, pp 207–219.
6. Munson P: Principles of Pharmacology. Basic Concepts and Clinical Applications, 1st ed. New York: Chapman and Hall, 1996, pp 1130–1133.
7. Hirsch J, Warkentin T, Raschke R, et al: Heparin and low-molecular-weight heparin: mechanisms of action, pharmacokinetics, dosing considerations, monitoring, efficacy, and safety. Cardiopulm Crit Care J 114: 489–510, 1998.
8. Hirsch J, Dalen J, Anderson DR et al: Oral anticoagulants: mechanisms of action, clinical effectiveness, and optimal therapeutic range. Cardiopulm Crit Care J 114:445–469, 1998.
9. Marion PL: The ICU Book, 2nd ed. Baltimore: Williams & Wilkins, 1998.
10. Porche R, Brenner ZR: Allergy to protamine sulfate. Heart Lung J Acute Crit Care 28:418–428, 1999.
11. Franz MG: Use of the wound healing trajectory as an outcome determinant for acute wound healing. Wound Repair Regen 8:511–516, 2000.
12. Youn B: Oxygen and Its Role in Wound Healing. Hyperbarics, Environmental Tectonics Corporation, 2000.
13. Rosito GB: Diagnosis of coagulation disorders. Cardiol Clin 14:239–250, 1996.
14. Fauci AS: Harrinson's Principles of Internal Medicine, 14th ed. New York: McGraw-Hill, 1998.
15. Cotran RS: Robbins Pathologic Basis of Disease, 6th ed. Philadelphia: WB Saunders, 1999.
16. O'Leary JP: The Physiologic Basis of Surgery, 2nd ed. Baltimore: Williams & Wilkins, 1996.

NOTES

Immunology and Infection

QUESTIONS

1. Toxic epidermal necrolysis related to drugs is potentially a serious problem because of the established overall mortality rate of 25% to 50%, which is related to fluid and electrolyte problems and secondary infections. In the United States, which drug is the most common cause of this disease?
   a. Phenobarbital
   b. Bactrim
   c. Metronidazole
   d. Warfarin
   e. Phenytoin

2. A 55-year-old diabetic white woman who is allergic to penicillin undergoes right hemicolectomy for colon cancer. Twelve hours after surgery, she complains of excruciating pain at the incision site. On physical examination, the wound shows swelling, erythema, and an advancing edge with brownish skin discoloration. A thin brown discharge is present. A smear is taken with identification of a gram-positive organism. Repeat examination after 3 hours shows progression of the discoloration and bleb formation. The most appropriate antibiotic for this condition would be:
   a. Cefazolin
   b. Azithromycin
   c. Clindamycin

d. Aztreonam
e. Levofloxacin

3. A 25-year-old man presents with 25% partial-thickness burns. During the course of his hospitalization, Sulfamylon burn cream is used to treat his wound infection. Which of the following statements is correct regarding this agent?
   a. It is bactericidal.
   b. It is poorly diffusible with suboptimal eschar penetration.
   c. It produces no pain when applied to partial-thickness burns.
   d. It inhibits the enzyme carbonic anhydrase.
   e. It causes neutropenia.

4. The most common mechanism by which antibiotic resistance is mediated is:
   a. Enzymatic inhibition (the antibiotic is destroyed by chemical modification by an enzyme that is elaborated by the resistant bacteria)
   b. Altered porin channels
   c. Alterations of outer or inner membrane permeability
   d. Alteration of target proteins (the target structure in the bacterium can be reprogrammed to have a low affinity for antibiotic recognition)
   e. Antibiotic efflux (the drug is pumped out faster than it can diffuse in, so intrabacterial concentrations are kept low and ineffectual)

5. Regarding B lymphocytes, which of the following statements is true?
   a. B lymphocytes account for 30% to 40% of the circulating pool of lymphocytes.
   b. The majority of these cells expresses IgG and IgM on their surface.
   c. The majority of these cells do not carry MHC class II antigens.

d. Plasma cells are the final product of B-cell clonal selection and express complement receptor in their surface.
e. CD20 antigen is expressed on resting and activated B lymphocytes.

6. Regarding antibiotic therapy, which of the following statements is correct?
   a. Tetracyclines can produce the syndrome of inappropriate antidiuretic hormone.
   b. Clindamycin, a bactericidal antibiotic, has a good spectrum of activity with gram-positive organisms and anaerobes.
   c. Penicillins acts by inhibition of transpeptidases and carboxypeptidases, necessary enzymes for the cross-linking of the cell wall.
   d. Quinolones have a good distribution, including bone and cerebral spinal fluid.
   e. Amphotericin B should be infused centrally; side effects including liver failure and hyperkalemia are not uncommon.

7. Regarding *Actinomyces israelii*, which one of the following statements is incorrect?
   a. It is an anaerobic gram-positive branching rod.
   b. It is not found, unless pathologically, in the normal human flora.
   c. Toxin or virulence factors are not known.
   d. It can cause abscesses with sulfur granules in exudates.
   e. It is susceptible to penicillin.

8. Regarding methicillin-resistant *Staphylococcus aureus* (MRSA), which one of the following statements is true?
   a. Patients colonized by MRSA do not require mandatory isolation.

b. The treatment of choice is quinupristin/dalfopristin or linezolid.
c. MRSA appears to be due to changes in major penicillin-binding proteins.
d. Endotoxin is the major agent responsible for MRSA pathogenicity.
e. MRSA is not found in the normal human flora.

9. Regarding *Bacteroides* species, which one of the following statements is correct?
   a. *Bacteroides* species are gram-positive rods.
   b. *Bacteroides* species are the second most common organisms in the colonic flora.
   c. *Bacteroides fragilis* is cultured in approximately 30% of intraperitoneal abscesses.
   d. They usually do not play any role in biliary stent occlusion.
   e. Succinic acid, produced by *Bacteroides* species and other anaerobes, may facilitate coinfection by other organisms because of inhibition of phagocytic cells.

10. Which is the organism most commonly associated with hematogenous osteomyelitis?
   a. *Salmonella*
   b. *Escherichia coli*
   c. *Staphylococcus aureus*
   d. *Streptococcus pyogenes*
   e. *Bacteroides*

ANSWERS

1. TOXIC EPIDERMAL NECROLYSIS: correct answer e

This severe cutaneous and systemic reaction may represent the most severe end of the spectrum of erythema multiforme major (or Stevens-Johnson syndrome). This eruption has been confused in the past with what is now called *staphylococcal scalded skin syndrome.* Toxic epidermal necrolysis should be used only for disease not related to *Staphylococcus* toxin. The onset of a morbilliform to diffuse, often generalized erythema is often preceded by several hours to days by skin tenderness, fever, malaise, and arthralgias. The skin resembles an extensive transepidermal burn. Tzank preparations, showing cuboidal cells, and skin biopsy can be used to confirm the diagnosis. A specific drug is implicated in 70% of cases. Phenytoin and phenobarbital are the leading causes in the United States, with other antibiotics and drugs such as allopurinol and nonsteroidal anti-inflammatory drugs (e.g., ibuprofen) following in frequency. Various nondrug causes, including graft-versus-host disease, infections, and neoplasms, have been implicated. Acute use of systemic steroids remains controversial. Toxic epidermal necrolysis remains a disease of severe morbidity and high mortality (25% to 50%).[1]

2. CLOSTRIDIAL GAS GANGRENE: correct answer c

Clostridial gas gangrene is produced by a gram-positive, spore-producing organism found both in the gastrointestinal tract of the individual and widely throughout nature. The most common invading organism is *Clostridium perfringens*, responsible in 80% to 90% of cases. The clostridial organism is not a strict anaerobe, as 30% mm Hg of oxygen allows free growth, whereas 70% mm Hg oxygen restricts growth. The spectrum of focal clostridial infection runs from insignificant wound contamination to deep myonecrosis, toxemia, and death. The major exotoxins causing spread of the disease are α-lecithinase C, collagenase, hyaluronidase, and fibrolysin. Vascular insufficiency, IV drug abuse, gastrointestinal surgery, and diabetes are important predisposing factors. Within hours of injury, the wound becomes swollen, painful, tender, and red or mottled. As the infection spreads along tissue planes, frank bullae, necrosis, and gangrene occur. The characteristic sign, crepitation due to gas in the tissues, may be elicited by pressure at the wound margin or demonstrated by radiography; however, neither is constant. Data support a striking association of *Clostridium septicum* infection with colorectal and hematologic malignancies and with immunosuppressed patients. Penicillin G in a dose of 20 million units/day in adults and 100,000 to 250,000 units/kg/day IV every 4 hours in children is the treatment of choice for serious infections. In case of penicillin allergy or concern about resistance, other antibiotics such as clindamycin, chloramphenicol, metronidazole, tetracycline, vancomycin, or imipenem should be considered. The overall mortality rate may be significantly reduced when prompt hyperbaric oxygen therapy is adjunctively used with appropriate antibiotics and surgical debridement.[2–4]

3. BURN WOUND CARE: correct answer d

Sulfamylon burn cream is an 11.1% suspension of mafenide acetate, which is bacteriostatic, freely soluble, and readily diffuses through the eschar to establish an effective concentration at the nonviable/viable tissue interface. This agent has the broadest spectrum against gram-negative organisms, particularly *Pseudomonas*. The principal limitations are the pain produced by its application to partial-thickness burns and its inhibition of carbonic anhydrase, which promotes wasting of bicarbonate by the kidney and accentuates postburn hyperventilation. Both of these derangements predispose the patient to acidosis.

Silver sulfadiazine (Silvadene) burn cream is bacteriostatic but poorly diffusible and penetrates the eschar less than mafenide acetate burn cream, produces no pain when applied to partial-thickness burns, and causes no electrolyte or acid-base disturbances. The principal limitations of these agents include the development of neutropenia and ineffectiveness against some gram-negative organisms (some *Pseudomonas* strains and virtually all *Enterobacter cloacae* organisms). Silver nitrate does not penetrate the eschar, and its principal limitation consists of the leaching of sodium, potassium, chloride, and calcium from the wound and the trans-eschar absorption of the aqueous vehicle, which may lead to mineral deficits, alkalosis, and water loading.[5]

4. GENERAL MECHANISMS OF ANTIBIOTIC RESISTANCE: correct answer a

Antimicrobial resistance is associated with high morbidity and mortality, high cost, and prolonged hospitalization. Higher morbidity and mortality rates may be associated with greater difficulty in clearing infections, a need for more invasive procedures to eradicate deep-seated infections, and higher relapse rates.

Bacteria evade antimicrobial action by adopting diverse mechanisms. These mechanisms include enzymatic inhibition, altered porin channels, alterations of outer or inner membrane permeability, alteration of target proteins, antibiotic efflux, and altered metabolic pathways (auxotrophs). Enzymatic inhibition is one of the most common modes of antimicrobial resistance and is usually mediated by plasmids. A principal mechanism for the rapid spread of antibiotic-resistance genes through bacterial populations is that such genes get collected on plasmids that are independently replicated within and passed between bacterial cells and species.[6, 7]

5. B LYMPHOCYTES: correct answer e

The number of B lymphocytes found in peripheral blood ranges from 5% to 15%. B cells usually express a different variety of antigens. The majority of B cells carry MHC class II antigens that are important for cooperative interactions with T cells. CD19, CD20, and CD22 are the main markers for B lymphocytes. CD20 usually is expressed in resting and activated B cells but is not found on hematopoietic stem cells, pro B cells, or plasma cells. This B cell marker appears late in the cell maturation and is involved in B cell activation. Monoclonal antibodies have been used in treatment of B-cell lymphoma for blocking CD20. The immunoglobulins usually expressed at the surface of B cells are IgM and IgD. Plasma cells are antibody-producing cells. Plasma cells develop from B lymphocytes and are large and spherical and stain blue with Wright's stain. Plasma cells do not express on their surface immunoglobulin or complement receptors, which distinguishes them from B lymphocytes.[8, 9]

6. ANTIBIOTICS: correct answer c

Tetracyclines, such as demeclocycline, doxycycline, minocycline, and tetracycline, can cause permanent discoloration of teeth if used in children. Other side effects are phototoxicity, hepatotoxicity, and nephrogenic diabetes insipidus. Demeclocycline can be used to treat the syndrome of inappropriate antidiuretic hormone.

Clindamycin is a bacteriostatic antibiotic and indeed has a good spectrum of activity with gram-positive organisms and anaerobes.

Quinolone, an antibiotic that inhibits DNA gyrase (topoisomerase II) in bacteria, has good penetration in different tissues except cerebrospinal fluid. Amphotericin B can cause renal failure, renal tubular acidosis, hypokalemia, and hypomagnesemia.[10, 11]

7. INFECTIOUS DISEASE: correct answer b

Actinomyces israelii is an anaerobic gram-positive branching rod found in the normal flora of the mouth, colon, and female genital tract. Its virulence factors have not been well established. Actinomycosis presents with hard, nonpainful draining abscesses with grains (sulfur granules), which can be microscopic or macroscopic. *Actinomyces* has a tendency to cross anatomic boundaries, forming sinus tract fistulas. *Actinomyces* can be present in cervical infections (associated with intrauterine devices) and cervicofacial, thoracic, abdominal, and central nervous system abscesses. Classic disease is characterized by a densely fibrotic lesion that undergoes slow contiguous spread and ignores tissue planes.

Treatment consists of incision and drainage of the abscess. When antibiotic therapy is necessary, penicillin is the antibiotic of choice.[10]

8. INFECTIOUS DISEASE: correct answer c

MRSA resistance is mainly due to changes in the major penicillin-binding sites.

MRSA becomes resistant to methicillin by the acquisition of a chromosomal *mecA* gene, which encodes an alternative supplementary target called PBP 2a (or PBP 2) that has low affinity for β-lactams. Resistance to other antibiotics is mediated primarily through plasmids.

Careful, repeated, and compulsive hand washing should be a daily routine for hospital personnel and is of utmost importance. Patients with a history of MRSA infection should be strictly isolated.

MRSA pathogenicity is due to numerous exotoxins. Gram-positive cocci do not have endotoxins.

Patients with MRSA infection should be treated with vancomycin. Reports have shown MRSA strains resistant to vancomycin. Linezolid and quinupristin/dalfopristin may be effective when resistance is present.

Normal flora of the skin and nose harbor MRSA. A study showed that up to 70% of health care professionals and up to 30% of the general population have positive nose cultures for MRSA.[10, 12]

9. INFECTIOUS DISEASE: correct answer e

The virulence of *Bacteroides* species is due to the production of the short-chain fatty acid succinic acid, which inhibits phagocytosis, and may facilitate coinfection by other organisms.

The virulence is also due to a polysaccharide carbohydrate capsule that promotes abscess formation, pili and fimbriae (which facilitate epithelial adherence), and enzymatic action, including hyaluronidase, hemolysin, peroxidase, collagenase, phospholipase, protease, fibrinolysin, heparinase, and neuraminidase (which cause tissue necrosis and promote tissue invasion).

Bacteroides species are anaerobic gram-negative rods and are the most common bacteria in the colonic flora.

Bacteroides fragilis plays an important role in intra-abdominal infection, being cultured in 90% of cases. *Bacteroides fragilis* has been shown to play an important role in the occlusion of biliary stents as well.[10, 13, 14]

10. MICROBIOLOGY: correct answer c

Staphylococcus aureus is the most common organism in all age groups. Group B *Streptococcus* is a common organism in neonates, *Salmonella* is encountered in patients with sickle cell disease, and *Haemophilus influenzae* is a frequent organism associated with osteomyelitis in toddlers.[15, 16]

Quick Answers

1. E	6. C
2. C	7. B
3. D	8. C
4. A	9. E
5. E	10. C

R E F E R E N C E S

1. Moschella S, Hurley H: Dermatology, 3rd ed. Philadelphia: WB Saunders, 1992, pp 557, 583–584.
2. Cameron J: Current Surgical Therapy, 5th ed. St. Louis: CV Mosby, 1995, pp 913–914.
3. Moschella S, Hurley H: Dermatology, 3rd ed. Pennsylvania: Saunders,1992:772–773.
4. Yu V, Meringun T: Antimicrobial Therapy and Vaccines, 1st ed. Baltimore: Williams & Wilkins, 1999, pp 146–147.
5. Sabiston D: The Biological Basis of Modern Surgical Practice, 15th ed. Philadelphia: WB Saunders, 1997, pp 207–234.
6. Virk A, Steckelberg JM: Clinical aspects of antimicrobial resistance. Mayo Clin Proc 75:200–214, 2000.

7. Walsh C: Molecular mechanisms that confer antibacterial drug resistance. Nature 406:775–781, 2000.
8. Cruse JM, Lewis RE: Illustrated Dictionary of Immunology, 1st ed. Boca Raton: CRC Press, 1995.
9. Roitt IM, Brostaff J, Male DK: Immunology, 3rd ed. London: CV Mosby, 1993.
10. Mandell GL, Bennett JE, Dolin R: Principles and Practice of Infectious Disease, 5th ed. Philadelphia: Churchill Livingstone, 2000.
11. Gilman AG, Rall TW, Nies AS, Taylor P: The Pharmacologic Basis of Therapeutics, 8th ed. New York: Pergamon Press, 1990.
12. Bodi M: Impact of gram-positive resistance on outcome of nosocomial pneumonia. Crit Care Med 29(4 Suppl), 2001.
13. Leung JW: Early attachment of anaerobic bacteria may play an important role in biliary stent blockage. Gastrointest Endosc 52:725–729, 2000.
14. Townsend CM, Beauchamp RD, Evers BM, Mattox K: Sabiston Textbook of Surgery, 16th ed. Philadelphia: WB Saunders, 2001.
15. Behrman RE: Nelson Textbook of Pediatrics, 16th ed. Philadelphia: WB Saunders, 2000.
16. Canale ST: Campbell's Operative Orthopaedics, 9th ed. St. Louis: CV Mosby, 1998.

NOTES

Oncology

QUESTIONS

1. Which of the following is *not* a recommendation for early detection of cancer in an average-risk, asymptomatic person?
   a. In women, breast self-examination monthly after age 20 and annual mammography after age 40
   b. In men older than 50, annual digital examination and prostate-specific antigen (PSA) assay
   c. In men and women, cancer-related checkup every 3 years at ages 20 to 39 and annually after age 40
   d. Annual Papanicolaou (Pap) test and pelvic examination in all women who are or have been sexually active or who are 18 years or older
   e. Annual fecal occult blood test in men and women beginning at age 50 and flexible sigmoidoscopy every 3 years beginning at age 50
2. The major source of fuel of tumor cells comes from:
   a. Free fatty acids
   b. Glycogenolysis and acetyl CoA
   c. Ketone bodies, triglycerides, and glucose
   d. Glycolysis and glutaminolysis
   e. Is the same as normal cells
3. Which of the following genes is associated with the development of colon cancer?
   a. Carcinoembryonic antigen (CEA)

b. c-*myc*
c. Rb-1
d. p53
e. c-*erb*

4. Medullary thyroid carcinoma as part of the multiple endocrine neoplasia syndrome is associated with a mutation of which oncogene?
   a. k-*ras*
   b. RET
   c. p53
   d. her-2
   e. *myc*

5. Which of the following serum markers has the highest sensitivity/specificity for screening patients with a clinically occult malignancy?
   a. CA-125
   b. β-HCG
   c. PSA
   d. α-Fetoprotein
   e. CEA (carcinoembryonic antigen)

6. Tumor necrosis factor α is produced by:
   a. Fibroblasts
   b. Platelets
   c. Endothelial cells
   d. Macrophages
   e. Neutrophils

7. Where in the cell cycle does the tumor suppressor gene p53 prevent tumor cells from completing its replication?
   a. From mitosis to G_1 phase
   b. From G_1 to S phase
   c. From S to G_2 phase
   d. From G_2 to mitosis
   e. From G_1 to G_0 phase

8. All of the following are risk factors for endometrial cancer, except:
   a. Diabetes
   b. Late menopause
   c. Exogenous estrogen use
   d. Chronic anovulatory states
   e. Multiparity

9. A 49-year-old man underwent his last chemotherapy session for testicular cancer 3 weeks ago and now is complaining of shortness of breath. Which of the following drugs is most probably causing his problem?
   a. Doxorubicin (Adriamycin)
   b. Etoposide
   c. Streptozocin
   d. Bleomycin
   e. Vincristine

ANSWERS

1. CANCER SCREENING AND EARLY DETECTION: correct answer e

The American Cancer Society endorses the guidelines shown. A triad of early detection tests is recommended for persons at average risk: digital rectal examination, fecal occult blood test, and sigmoidoscopy. Digital rectal examination is recommended annually in patients older than 40. For the fecal occult blood test to be effective, persons with a positive result must be followed up appropriately (examination of the entire bowel by barium enema and sigmoidoscopy or total colonoscopy).

Flexible sigmoidoscopy should be performed every 5 years in men and women beginning at age 50.[1, 2]

2. TUMOR CELL BIOLOGY: correct answer d

Application of the quantitative theory of metabolic control of branched pathways provides a hypothesis to account for the high rate of both glycolysis and glutaminolysis in tumor cells. They provide metabolic intermediates for the synthesis of purine and pyrimidine nucleotides. In neoplastic cells, the action of glutaminase is similar to or greater than that of hexokinase, which suggests that glutamine may be as important as glucose for energy generation in these cells.[3]

3. GENETIC CHANGES IN COLON CANCER: correct answer d

Colon carcinoma is particularly suitable for the study of tumor progression because it develops slowly over several years and progresses through cytologically distinct benign and malignant stages of growth. A mutation that involves a predisposing gene called APC (adenomatous polyposis coli) on chromosome 5p transforms normal epithelial tissue lining the gut to hyperproliferating tissue. Activation of the Kristen *ras* (k-*ras*) proto-oncogene and loss of the DCC (deleted in colon cancer) gene are involved in the progression to a benign adenoma. Loss of the p53 gene and other chromosomal losses are involved in the progression to malignant carcinoma and metastasis. This sequence of events is not invariable, however, and may differ in some colon cancers. The p53 tumor suppressor gene is a frequent target for recessive mutations in many human malignancies and has been shown to initiate apoptosis in cells exposed to agents that cause DNA strand breakage, including gamma irradiation and various chemotherapeutic drugs. The product of the tumor suppressor gene p53 is a protein of 53 kd (hence the name).

The p53 protein prevents a cell from completing the cell cycle if its DNA is not properly replicated in S phase. It does this by binding to a transcription factor called E2F. The p53 protein has also been implicated in DNA repair.[4]

4. MEDULLARY THYROID CANCER: correct answer b

Twenty percent of medullary thyroid cancers (MTCs) are associated with familial patterns of occurrence. These include those cancers occurring in the setting of multiple endocrine neoplasia (MEN) types 2A and 2B and, less commonly, non-MEN familial MTC (FMTC). Recent studies have identified mutations in the RET proto-oncogene, which resides in the centromeric region of chromosome 10, in afflicted individuals in more than 90% of kindreds with MEN 2A and MEN 2B and approximately 70% of those with FMTC. RET is a tyrosine kinase receptor. These genetic findings have dramatically altered the approach to presymptomatic patients with MEN 2 and FMTC kindreds. Individuals related to patients with MTC in whom a mutation in the RET proto-oncogene has been detected are all screened for the RET mutation. Asymptomatic family members who carry the RET mutation are then offered prophylactic thyroidectomy. Thyroidectomy in children identified to be carriers of the RET mutation is recommended at age 5 years or thereafter once the diagnosis is made. In persons considered negative for the RET mutation by mutational analysis, the risk of MTC is thought to be essentially the same risk as for the general population, and thus no further evaluation is warranted.[5]

5. SERUM MARKERS: correct answer c

PSA is a serine protease produced by benign and malignant prostate epithelium. PSA is prostate-specific but not cancer-specific. Prostatitis, benign prostatic hypertrophy, and prostate manipulation can all cause an elevation of PSA. The serum half-life of PSA is approximately 3 days. Currently, PSA is the only serum marker with Food and Drug Administration (FDA) approval for the screening and early detection of prostate cancer. It is important to recognize that as men age, PSA levels increase owing to benign prostatic hypertrophy; therefore, many experts prefer to use age-adjusted PSA. Serum PSA also helps in defining the extent of disease. There is a clear-cut relation between the PSA level and the cancer stage.[6]

6. IMMUNOLOGY: correct answer d

After endotoxin exposure, macrophages are stimulated to produce tumor necrosis factor α, which mediates many of the systemic responses associated with infection. The target tissues–cells are endothelial cells, monocytes–macrophages, neutrophils, fibroblasts, and receptors in liver, muscle, lung, gut, and kidney. Tumor necrosis factor is also produced by lymphocytes, natural killer cells, glial cells, and Kupffer cells.[7]

7. p53 TUMOR SUPPRESSOR GENE: correct answer b

The normal p53 gene prevents the propagation of cells with damaged DNA by inducing cell cycle arrest until DNA can be repaired or by destroying the cell through apoptosis. The p53 gene induces transcription of the WAF1/Cipl gene, which produces a protein that binds to and sequesters cyclin-kinase complexes (cyclin E, CDK2) that are essential for cell cycle progression. This results in G_1 cell cycle arrest.[8]

8. ENDOMETRIAL CANCER: correct answer e

Risk factors for endometrial cancer include prolonged estrogenic stimulation, high doses of estrogen replacement therapy for menopausal symptoms, obesity, diabetes, hypertension, late first pregnancy, polycystic ovary disease, estrogen-secreting ovarian tumors, hypothyroidism, chronic anovulatory states, and low parity.[9]

9. ANTINEOPLASTIC AGENTS, SIDE EFFECTS: correct answer d

Doxorubicin may cause bone marrow suppression, alopecia, and cardiomyopathy.
Etoposide may cause alopecia, hepatotoxicity, diarrhea, and bone marrow suppression.
Streptozocin causes kidney toxicity and hyperglycemia.
Vincristine causes peripheral neuropathy, constipation, and alopecia.
Cisplatin has a high incidence of renal toxicity.
Cyclophosphamide may cause hemorrhagic cystitis.
Procarbazine may produce hypertension.
L-Asparaginase may produce acute pancreatitis.
Bleomycin may cause pulmonary toxicity (pneumonitis, fibrosis) and hyperpigmentation.[10, 11]

Quick Answers

1. E	4. B	7. B
2. D	5. C	8. E
3. D	6. D	9. D

REFERENCES

1. Murphy G: Clinical Oncology, 2nd ed. Atlanta: American Cancer Society, 1995, pp 181–191.
2. Holland J, Frei E: Cancer Medicine, 5th ed. Hamilton: American Cancer Society, 2000, p 368.
3. Newsholme EA, Board M: Application of metabolic control logic to fuel utilization and its significance in tumor cells. Adv Enzyme Reg 31:225–246, 1991.
4. Tannock I, Hill R: The Basic Science of Oncology, 3rd ed. New York: McGraw-Hill, 1998, pp 74–75, 101.
5. Sabiston D: The Biological Basis of Modern Surgical Practice, 15th ed. Philadelphia: WB Saunders, 1997, pp 30–31.
6. Bitran J: Expert Guide to Oncology, 1st ed. Philadelphia: American College of Physicians, 2000, pp 37–43.
7. Sabiston D: The Biological Basis of Modern Surgical Practice, 15th ed. Philadelphia: WB Saunders, 1997, pp 59–60.
8. Tannock I, Hill R: The Basic Science of Oncology, 3rd ed. New York: McGraw-Hill, 1998, pp 74–75, 101–102.
9. Sabiston D: The Biological Basis of Modern Surgical Practice, 15th ed. Philadelphia: WB Saunders, 1997.
10. Gilman AG, Rall TW, Nies AS, et al: The Pharmacologic Basis of Therapeutics, 8th ed. New York: Pergamon Press, 1990.
11. Leenhard R: Clinical Oncology, 1st ed. Atlanta: American Cancer Society, 2001.

NOTES

PART TWO

Clinical Science

Upper Gastrointestinal Tract (Æsophagus, Stomach, Duodenum, Hepatobiliary, and Pancreas)

QUESTIONS

1. A 33-year-old female (G1P0) at 15 weeks' gestation presents with a 2-day history of increasing right upper quadrant pain, nausea, and vomiting. Her temperature was 99.4°F and her white blood cell count was 19,800/mm^3 with 87% polymorphocytes and 5% bands. Other laboratory values were normal. The abdominal sonogram showed a distended gallbladder with a thickened wall and a stone impacted in the gallbladder neck. On the day of admission, the patient underwent laparoscopic cholecystectomy under general anesthesia. Regarding intraoperative management, all of the following are recommended and true except:
   a. Use of the Hasson open approach to establish the initial pneumoperitoneum
   b. Use of transvaginal ultrasonography rather than transabdominal ultrasonography if intraoperative monitoring is to be used
   c. Routine use of prophylactic tocolytic agents
   d. Use of compression stockings

e. Compared with open cholecystectomy, a laparoscopic approach decreases the risk of spontaneous abortion in the first trimester and preterm labor in the third trimester

2. Which of the following entities is the most common cause of upper gastrointestinal (GI) bleeding in patients infected with HIV-1?
   a. Kaposi sarcoma
   b. Cytomegalovirus gastritis
   c. Gastric lymphoma (non-Hodgkin)
   d. Gastric ulcers
   e. Stress ulcers

3. All of the following arteries supply the greater curvature of the stomach except:
   a. Splenic artery
   b. Left gastroepiploic artery
   c. Gastroduodenal artery
   d. Left gastric artery
   e. Right gastroepiploic artery

4. The management and surgical approach of GI stromal tumors include all of the following characteristics except:
   a. The most powerful prognostic indicator is tumor size and necrosis.
   b. Recent studies show that CD34 marker–positive GI stromal tumors frequently do not show evidence of smooth muscle differentiation.
   c. Acute GI hemorrhage is the initial presentation of gastric GI stromal tumors in more than 50% of patients with no previous symptoms.
   d. Malignant GI stromal tumors have a low propensity for intramural extension.
   e. Lymphadenectomy is not necessary unless the lymph nodes are grossly involved.

5. The second most common site of gastrinomas, after the pancreas, is the:
   a. Stomach
   b. Duodenum
   c. Jejunum
   d. Ileum
   e. Retroperitoneum
6. Which of the following intestinal segments yields the best autograft for total esophageal replacement?
   a. Ascending colon
   b. Transverse colon
   c. Descending colon
   d. Ileocolon
   e. Sigmoid colon
7. A 75-year-old woman with no previous history of abdominal surgery presents with intermittent cramping abdominal pain, abdominal distention, nausea, and vomiting. Plain films of the abdomen show distended loops of bowel and air in the biliary tree. Regarding this pathologic process:
   a. Stones may become impacted in the descending colon, the narrowest portion of the colon.
   b. Bouveret syndrome occurs when there is an impacted stone in the jejunum.
   c. The intestinal obstruction is life-threatening and must be treated urgently.
   d. The overall mortality rate is approximately 50%.
   e. Cholecystenteric fistula rarely closes spontaneously.
8. A 3-year-old boy presents with abdominal pain, jaundice, and a palpable abdominal mass in the right upper quadrant. The initial work-up for

jaundice reveals mildly increased hepatic transaminase levels and significantly increased alkaline phosphatase, γ-glutamyl transferase, and bilirubin levels. Ultrasonographic imaging shows a cystic dilatation of the bile ducts. Subsequently, endoscopic retrograde cholangiopancreatography shows a fusiform dilatation of the extrahepatic biliary tree. What is the best treatment option for this child and what is the most serious complication of this condition?

a. Cyst excision; cholangitis
b. Cyst excision; bile duct cancer
c. Complete cyst resection; cholangitis
d. Cyst excision; liver failure
e. Complete cyst excision with Roux-en-Y hepaticojejunostomy; bile duct cancer

9. Regarding location, size, malignant potential, and multiplicity, the statement that best describes insulinomas is:
   a. Head of the pancreas, >5 cm, malignant, and single
   b. Uncinate process, <2 cm, benign, and single
   c. Pancreas, >5 cm, malignant, and multiple
   d. Uniformly distributed throughout the pancreas (head, body, tail), <2 cm, benign, and single
   e. Body of the pancreas, <2 cm, malignant, and multiple

10. A 45-year-old man presents with epigastric abdominal pain and intermittent nausea and vomiting. Past surgical history reveals a Billroth II gastrojejunostomy performed 5 years before. Endoscopy reveals a beefy red appearance to the gastric mucosa. Gastric emptying results are normal. What surgical procedure is indicated for this condition?

a. Total gastrectomy with Roux-en-Y esophagojejunostomy
b. Conversion to Billroth I gastroduodenostomy
c. Antiperistaltic reversed jejunal segment
d. Roux-en-Y biliary diversion
e. Isoperistaltic jejunal interposition

11. With laparoscopic Nissen fundoplication, the correct intraoperative sequence of events should be:
    a. Division of the hepatogastric ligament, dissection of the crura and phrenoesophageal ligament, lengthening of the abdominal esophagus-retroesophageal dissection at the gastroesophageal (GE) junction, bougie placement, closure of the esophageal hiatus, retroesophageal wrap, fixation of the wrap to the right crus
    b. Division of the hepatogastric ligament, dissection of the crura and phrenoesophageal ligament, bougie placement, lengthening of the abdominal esophagus, retroesophageal dissection at the GE junction, closure of the esophageal hiatus, retroesophageal wrap, fixation of the wrap to the right crus
    c. Division of the hepatogastric ligament, dissection of the crura and phrenoesophageal ligament, lengthening of the abdominal esophagus, retroesophageal dissection at the GE junction, bougie placement, retroesophageal wrap, closure of the esophageal hiatus, fixation of the wrap to the right crus
    d. Dissection of the crura and phrenoesophageal ligament, division of the hepatogastric ligament, lengthening of the abdominal esophagus, retroesophageal dissection at the GE junction, bougie

placement, closure of the esophageal hiatus, retroesophageal wrap, fixation of the wrap to the right crus

e. Dissection of the crura and phreno-esophageal ligament, division of the hepato-gastric ligament, bougie placement, lengthening of the abdominal esophagus, retroesophageal dissection at the GE junction, closure of the esophageal hiatus, retroesophageal wrap, fixation of the wrap to the right crus

12. When performing a laparoscopic Nissen fundoplication for gastroesophageal reflux disease, the most common mechanisms of failure of the operation are:
    a. Transdiaphragmatic herniation of the fundoplication
    b. Slipped or misplaced wrap
    c. Twisted wrap
    d. Disruption of the wrap
    e. Wrap too long or too short

13. Which of the following statements about duodenal diverticular disease is not true?
    a. The duodenum is the second most common location for diverticula formation, after the sigmoid.
    b. Most extraluminal duodenal diverticula occur in the lateral wall of the second portion of the duodenum.
    c. More than 90% of cases are asymptomatic.
    d. Patients with symptomatic extraluminal duodenal diverticula should undergo nonsurgical treatment, unless complications occur.
    e. The most common complication is choledocholithiasis.

14. Which of the following hepatic lesions should be resected in the asymptomatic patient?
    a. 3-cm hepatic adenoma
    b. 5-cm focal nodular hyperplasia
    c. 6-cm hepatic hemangioma
    d. 4-cm hepatic hamartoma
    e. 2-cm hydatid cyst

15. Regarding gastric anatomy, physiology, and pathology, which of the following statements is correct?
    a. *Helicobacter pylori,* a gram-negative bacteria that produces urease, has been implicated in the genesis of gastric carcinoma.
    b. The right and left gastroepiploic arteries—branches of the gastroduodenal and left gastric arteries, respectively—are responsible for the blood supply of the greater curvature of the stomach.
    c. Truncal vagotomy accelerates emptying of solids and delays emptying of liquids.
    d. In patients with Zollinger-Ellison syndrome, the treatment of choice for multiple ulcers is total gastrectomy.
    e. Gastric cancers are the most common tumors in the GI tract to present with submucosal spreading, needing at least 5 cm of resection margins.

16. Regarding pancreatic anatomy, which of the following statements is correct?
    a. The pancreas has a rich blood supply, part of which is derived from the inferior mesenteric artery.
    b. In 60% of cases, the ducts of Wirsung and Santorini open into the duodenum independently.

c. In 30% of cases, the duct of Santorini carries the entire secretion of the pancreas and the duct of Wirsung ends blindly.
d. The body of the pancreas lies to the right of the superior mesenteric artery and is related to the fourth portion of the duodenum.
e. The uncinate process is located anterior to the superior mesenteric artery.

17. Regarding hemobilia, which one of the following statements is correct?
    a. Gallstones constitute the most important cause of hemobilia.
    b. The most common tumor to cause hemobilia is hepatoblastoma.
    c. Hemobilia always presents as an acute onset of upper or lower GI bleeding.
    d. A red blood cell scan is considered the gold standard for the diagnosis of hemobilia.
    e. A false aneurysm within the parenchyma of the liver is best treated by embolization.

ANSWERS

1. GALLSTONE DISEASE DURING PREGNANCY: correct answer c

Pregnancy predisposes women to gallbladder disease because of hormonal changes that cause an increase in gallbladder volume during fasting, an increased residual volume after emptying, an increased saturation of bile with cholesterol, and a decreased circulating bile salt pool. Biliopancreatic disease during pregnancy is a relatively uncommon event that may affect 5 to 10 gravid women for every 10,000 deliveries. The frequency of choledocholithiasis in pregnancy requiring surgical intervention has been reported to be as low as 1 per 1200 deliveries. Most authors agree that surgery is indicated for complicated cases, such as refractory or recurrent biliary colic, acute cholecystitis, choledocholithiasis, and gallstone pancreatitis. Conservative medical management of these disorders has been shown to be unsuccessful in a high percentage of cases, requiring multiple admissions for recurrent symptoms. Most pregnant women respond to initial medical management; however, 70% experience relapse and, of these, 90% require hospitalization. The risk of relapse after successful initial medical management is 92% in women who present during the first trimester, 64% in women who present during the second trimester, and 44% in women who present during the third trimester. When symptomatic biliary disease occurs early in pregnancy, it is preferable to postpone surgery until the second trimester. Likewise, third-trimester disease is managed conservatively until the immediate postpartum period. It is generally agreed that any patient whose condition deteriorates while being treated medically should undergo emergent surgery regardless of the trimester.[1]

If intraoperative monitoring is to be used, transvaginal ultrasonography is preferred over transabdominal ultrasonography because the former provides continuous fetal heart rate monitoring, can be obtained with a minimal risk of contamination of the operative field, and the signal is not compromised by the pneumoperitoneum. There is no evidence to support the routine use of prophylactic tocolytic agents; they are rarely necessary and are associated with significant side effects. The risk of thromboembolic complications is increased in pregnancy. Pregnancy is associated with increased levels of fibrinogen and factors VII and XII, as well as a decrease in antithrombin III. In addition, uterine compression on the inferior vena cava, increased intra-abdominal pressure from insufflation, use of the reverse Trendelenburg position during laparoscopic surgery, and side effects of anesthesia all contribute to decreased venous return and an increased risk of deep venous thrombosis. For these reasons, the use of antiembolic measures is critical: Rapid mobilization, heparin (5000 U subcutaneously twice a day), and compression stockings are recommended.[2]

2. SURGICAL ASPECTS OF AIDS: correct answer a

Pathology due to HIV-1 infection affecting the stomach and duodenum usually presents with symptoms of abdominal pain, bleeding, gastric outlet obstruction, or perforation. The most common cause of upper GI bleeding in HIV-1–infected patients is Kaposi sarcoma.[3]

3. ANATOMY OF THE STOMACH: correct answer d

The arterial supply of the stomach comes mostly from the celiac system. The celiac artery sends branches to the lesser curve (left gastric and right gastric arteries) and to the greater curve (splenic, short gastric, gastroduodenal, left gastroepiploic, and right gastroepiploic arteries).[4]

4. GASTROINTESTINAL STROMAL TUMORS: correct answer a

Gastrointestinal stromal tumors are a group of intramural intestinal tumors formerly called *leiomyomas* or *leiomyosarcomas*. Recent pathology studies have shown that CD34 marker–positive GI stromal tumors frequently lack evidence of smooth muscle differentiation. Hence, it is suggested that these tumors be called *GI stromal tumors* rather than *smooth muscle tumors of the GI tract*. The most powerful prognostic indicator is the mitotic count (the number of mitotic figures found in a specified number of high-power fields). Other factors are less accurate. Gastric malignancies are of stromal origin in 1% to 2% of cases. In contrast with adenocarcinoma of the stomach, the initial presentation of gastric GI stromal tumors is often an acute upper GI hemorrhage with no previous symptoms. Malignant GI stromal tumors have a low propensity for intramural extension. Margins of only 1 to 2 cm are required because of the minimal extension. Lymphadenectomy is not necessary unless the lymph nodes are grossly involved, which is rare. A review of published series gave nodal metastasis rates of 7% to 13%. The same principle applies to the adjacent organs. They should not be included in the resection because they are usually isolated from the tumor by the pseudocapsule and not connected by tumor invasion or encasement. The reported rate of metastatic spread is between 3% and 38%.

The main problem in the asymptomatic patient is to determine whether or not the stromal cell tumor has malignant potential, and this is not always shown by histologic analysis.[5]

Endoscopic ultrasonography is reliable in predicting the potential malignancy of GI stromal tumors. The three most predictive endoscopic ultrasonography features are irregular margins, cystic spaces, and lymph nodes with a malignant pattern. In a recent study, the presence of at least one of these criteria had a sensitivity of 91%, a specificity of 88%, a positive predictive value of 83%, and a negative predictive value of 94% for potential malignancy. A combination of two of these three criteria had a positive predictive value and specificity of 100%.[6]

5. GASTRINOMAS: correct answer b

Duodenal gastrinomas are typically submucosal; 85% of gastrinomas occur in the "gastrinoma triangle," an anatomic area bounded by the junction of the cystic and common bile ducts superiorly, the junction of the second and third portions of the duodenum inferiorly, and the junction of the neck and body of the pancreas medially.[7, 8]

6. GASTROINTESTINAL AUTOGRAFTS: correct answer c

The ascending colon, transverse colon, descending colon, and ileocolon have all been used for autografts. The ileocecal valve continues to function as a partially competent valve after transplantation, thus preventing reflux up the ileal component of the graft. However, the descending colon has a better diameter, a more muscular and a less distensible wall, and a more dependable blood supply for total esophageal replacement than any other segment of large bowel. Whether based on the left colic artery to produce an isoperistaltic graft or based on the middle colic artery to produce an antiperistaltic tube, the large marginal artery ensures adequate perfusion.[9]

7. GALLSTONE ILEUS: correct answer c

Gallstone ileus has a higher incidence in females (3:1), and the average age of presentation is 72 years. Erosion of a gallstone through the gallbladder wall and subsequently through the wall of the small bowel or colon, leading to intestinal obstruction, is the usual sequence of events. The duodenum, the hepatic flexure of the colon, and the jejunum are the segments of intestine most commonly involved. Usually, the stone becomes impacted in the ileum, the narrowest portion of the small bowel. Another frequent site of impaction is the sigmoid, the narrowest portion of the colon.

Diagnosis is based on clinical findings and diagnostic studies. The classic findings in plain films are air in the biliary tree, distended loops of bowel, and an opaque gallstone in the small bowel or colon. Impacted stones are visible in 20% of cases; air in the biliary tree can be seen in 40%.

Bouveret syndrome occurs when a gallstone becomes impacted in the duodenum. Patients present with nausea and vomiting but no cramping or abdominal distention.

Treatment of gallstone ileus results in immediate relief of the bowel obstruction. Studies have shown that concomitant treatment of the bowel obstruction and cholecystenteric fistula increase morbidity and mortality. Moreover, cholecystenteric fistula closes spontaneously in many patients.[10]

The mortality of gallstone ileus ranges from 5% to 20%. Many factors contribute to this high mortality rate, which includes the elderly population affected, delayed diagnosis, and the presence of two concomitant pathologic processes (bowel obstruction and biliary fistula).[11]

8. BILE DUCT CYSTS: correct answer e

Cystic disorders of the bile ducts are most commonly diagnosed in children (80%). Few patients show the supposedly classic triad of jaundice, abdominal pain, and abdominal mass. The disease presents as a biliary obstructive process with increased γ-glutamyl transferase, alkaline phosphatase, and bilirubin.

The initial imaging test of choice is ultrasonography in children and computed tomography in adults. More detailed imaging information should be obtained with endoscopic retrograde cholangiopancreatography.

Complications associated with bile cystic disease include cholangitis, pancreatitis, biliary stones, and biliary cirrhosis. The most serious complication is bile duct cancer. The risk of malignancy is increased 12-fold in patients treated with a nonresection operation.[10, 11] Treatment is individualized according the bile cyst diverticulum type as shown in Table 6–1.

9. INSULINOMAS: correct answer d

Insulinomas are usually benign tumors, measuring less than 2 cm and uniformly distributed throughout the pancreatic tissue. Preoperative radiologic imaging is not usually successful in demonstrating the location of the tumor itself. A calcium angiogram, wherein calcium is selectively injected into the splenic artery, can identify the affected region of the pancreas. Interestingly enough, many studies have shown that intraoperative ultrasonography can identify these tumors. Furthermore,

TABLE 6—1

Title

	Description	**Treatment**
Type I	Fusiform dilatation of the extrahepatic biliary duct	Complete cyst excision with Roux-en-Y
Type II	Diverticulum of the extrahepatic biliary duct	Excision with primary choledochorrhaphy
Type III	Dilatation of the intraduodenal portion CBD	Transduodenal cyst excision
Type IV	Multiple intrahepatic and extrahepatic bile duct cysts	Selective management
Type V	Single or multiple intrahepatic biliary cysts	Selective management

intraoperative ultrasonography can help in safe enucleation of insulinomas, demonstrating the relation of these tumors with the pancreatic duct.[11, 12]

10. ALKALINE REFLUX GASTRITIS: correct answer d

Alkaline reflux is associated with burning epigastric pain, nausea, and bilious vomit. It is important to differentiate this condition from other postvagotomy syndromes.

Upper GI endoscopy shows variable degrees of acute and chronic gastritis and allows identification of other conditions, such as marginal anastomotic ulceration, afferent loop syndrome, and anastomotic stricture. Gastric emptying studies should be performed because gastroparesis can mimic some aspects of alkaline reflux.

Roux-en-Y biliary diversion has been the surgical treatment of choice. Creation of a 50-cm Roux-en-Y limb adequately diverts almost all afferent limb secretions away from the stomach.

Conversion of Billroth II to Billroth I gastroenterostomy and an interpositional jejunal loop are surgical procedures indicated for the treatment of dumping syndrome after partial gastrectomy.[11, 13, 14]

11. LAPAROSCOPIC FUNDOPLICATION: correct answer a

The correct sequence should be as follows:

1. Positioning and trocar placement
2. Liver retraction
3. Division of the hepatogastric ligament
4. Dissection of the crura and phrenoesophageal ligament
5. Lengthening of the abdominal esophagus (if necessary)

6. Stomach mobilization and ligation of short gastric vessels
7. Retroesophageal dissection at the gastroesophageal junction
8. Bougie placement
9. Closure of the esophageal hiatus
10. Retroesophageal wrap
11. Suture placement for wrap
12. Fixation of the wrap to right crus
13. Trocar removal[15]

12. LAPAROSCOPIC FUNDOPLICATION: correct answer a

Gastroesophageal fundoplication performed through a laparotomy or thoracotomy has a failure rate of 9% to 30% and requires revision in most patients who have recurrent or new foregut symptoms. The mechanism of failure is transdiaphragmatic herniation of the fundoplication in 41% of cases, followed by a slipped Nissen fundoplication in 16%.[16]

13. DUODENAL DIVERTICULA: correct answer b

Diverticula may occur anywhere, from the esophagus to the colon. A duodenal diverticulum is the most common small bowel diverticulum, followed by Meckel diverticulum. The duodenum is the second most common location after the sigmoid in the GI tract. There are two types: *extraluminal* (which usually are acquired) and *intraluminal* (which usually are congenital). The most common form is the extraluminal, false type. There is no gender predilection, and most extraluminal diverticula (>85%) occur in the second and medial portion of the duodenum within 2.5 cm of Vater's ampulla. These are called *prevaterian, juxtampullary,* or *periampullary*. The typical size is between 2 and 3 cm, and more than 90% of these diverticula are asymptomatic; only 1%

may require surgical intervention. The diagnosis is usually made as an incidental finding during laparotomy, endoscopy, or radiographic examination. If a diverticulum is suspected, a barium swallow or a hypotonic duodenography is indicated. The literature is consistent regarding nonsurgical management for patients with uncomplicated, symptomatic, extraluminal duodenal diverticula. The most common complications are choledocholithiasis, diverticulitis, bleeding, and stricture of the common bile duct or pancreatic duct. Perforation is rare (0.9% incidence). This is managed by kocherization of the duodenum, diverticulectomy near the neck, and primary closure. An omental patch should be placed over the repair. A feeding jejunostomy is also recommended. For the intraluminal type, the standard treatment is duodenotomy and excision.[17]

14. HEPATIC ADENOMAS: correct answer a

Benign Liver Lesions. Hepatic adenoma is a benign hepatocellular tumor strongly associated with the use of oral contraceptives. They also occur during pregnancy, in patients taking steroids or androgenic hormones, and in metabolic diseases such as diabetes mellitus and glycogen storage disease.

Hepatic adenoma is a well-circumscribed, often encapsulated, hypervascular tumor. Microscopically, hepatocytes rearrange in cords. Scintigraphic examination reveals no uptake. Conversely, computed tomography, magnetic resonance imaging, and angiography show peripheral enhancement of the lesion. Although regression and disappearance of hepatic adenomas have been reported after discontinuation of oral contraceptives, the potential for bleeding and malignant transformation, along with the current safety of hepatic surgery, favors routine resection.[18]

Focal Nodular Hyperplasia. Focal nodular hyperplasia is a benign hepatocellular lesion occurring most commonly in women (95%) of childbearing age. There is no established relation between oral contraceptives and focal nodular hyperplasia. The lesion has no true capsule, macroscopically shows a central stellate scar, and microscopically consists of hepatocytes and Kupffer cells separated by septa. On scintigraphic examination with technetium, the lesion takes up radioactive material because of the presence of Kupffer cells. Computed tomography with contrast shows a hyperdense lesion on the hepatic phase and an isodense lesion on the venous phase. Angiography reveals a hypervascular lesion with vessels evident in the central scar in a "spoke-wheel" pattern of enhancement. Resection is occasionally indicated if the patient is symptomatic.[19]

Hemangiomas are the most common lesions of the liver, women being affected more often than men. Hemangiomas are well-circumscribed lesions, usually less than 5 cm in the greater diameter and asymptomatic. Hemangiomas rarely rupture. Scintigraphic imaging with technetium-labeled red blood cells is virtually diagnostic if positive for hemangioma. Computed tomography, magnetic resonance imaging, and angiography show a centripetal and a peripheral enhancement. Pain, mass effect, platelet trapping, and early rupture are all indications for resection.

Hamartomas are composed of normal tissues rearranged in a disorganized fashion. When hamartomas are clinically significant, resection is indicated.

Small asymptomatic hydatid cysts are not an indication for surgery. Symptomatic cysts should be resected, and marsupialization should be performed.[20] See Table 6–2.

TABLE 6—2

Benign Liver Tumors

Lesion	Sex	Pathology	Imaging	Treatment
Hemangioma	F>M	Well-circumscribed mass composed of single endothelial layer	CT, MRI, angiocentripetal enhancement Scintigraphy + enhancement	Resection should be performed in symptomatic patients
Focal nodular hyperplasia	F>M	No true encapsulation, central stellate scar Hepatocytes/Kupffer cells separated by septa	CT hyperdense hepatic phase Angiography spoke-wheel Scintigraphy + enhancement	Resection should be performed in symptomatic patients
Hepatic adenoma	F>M	Encapsulated, cords of hepatocytes Scintigraphy with no enhancement	CT, MRI, angiography positive with peripheral enhancement transformation and bleeding	Resection always performed because of malignant

CT = computed tomography; MRI = magnetic resonance imaging.

15. STOMACH: correct answer a

Many factors have been implicated in the genesis of gastric cancer (GC). Diet—especially smoked, salty foods—and alcohol consumption have been associated with GC. GC is also associated with pernicious anemia, chronic atrophic gastritis, and reflux gastritis. GC is strongly associated with *Helicobacter pylori*; this association is based on the increase incidence of GC in areas with a high percentage of *H. pylori* infection in the United States.

The stomach has a rich blood supply. The lesser curvature of the stomach is supplied by the left gastric artery (branch of the celiac trunk). The greater curvature is vascularized by the right gastroepiploic artery, a branch of the gastroduodenal artery, and by the left gastroepiploic artery, a branch of the splenic artery. The right gastric artery originates from the common hepatic artery and supplies blood to the pyloroduodenal area. The short gastric arteries come from the splenic artery and supply blood to the fundus of the stomach.[21]

Regarding the physiology of the stomach, the fundus is responsible for emptying liquids, and the pyloroantral region is responsible for emptying solid particles. After a truncal vagotomy, the emptying of solids is delayed and the emptying of liquids is accelerated. Parietal cell vagotomy is associated only with increased emptying of liquids and no change in emptying of solids. Gastric resection procedures, such as the Billroth I and II procedures, also increases stomach emptying. Conversely, Roux-en-Y gastrojejunostomy results in a delay of stomach emptying.

Esophageal cancer is the most common GI tract tumor to present with submucosal spreading.

Ninety-five percent of GCs are adenocarcinomas. Lymphoma, carcinoids, leiomyosarcoma, and squamous cell carcinoma are the other frequent histologic types to involve the stomach. Adenocarcinoma can present as diffuse or intestinal. The latter type is usually well differentiated, forms glands, and is associated with metaplasia and chronic gastritis. The diffuse type is poorly differentiated, does not form glands, and is composed of signet ring cells. Nine percent of patients present with involvement of the entire stomach, known as *linitis plastica,* which carries a dismal prognosis.

Regarding the treatment of gastric ulcers in patients with Zollinger-Ellison syndrome, medical therapy with omeprazole is the first alternative. Truncal vagotomy and pyloroplasty or highly selective vagotomy are surgical options if medical therapy yields minimal relief.[11, 22]

16. PANCREATIC ANATOMY: correct answer b

The arterial blood supply of the head of the pancreas is derived from the branches of the gastroduodenal artery and superior mesenteric artery via anterior and posterior pancreaticoduodenal arcades. The body and tail of the pancreas are supplied from branches of the splenic artery and the superior mesenteric artery. The inferior mesenteric artery does not supply blood to the pancreatic gland.

In 60% of cases, the ducts of Wirsung and Santorini open into the duodenum independently. In 30% of cases, the duct of Wirsung carries the entire secretion of the pancreas and the duct of Santorini ends blindly. In 10% of cases, the duct of Santorini carries the entire pancreatic secretion and the duct of Wirsung is small or absent.[22, 23]

The body of the pancreas lies to the left of the superior mesenteric artery and is related to the fourth portion of the duodenum.

The uncinate process lies dorsal to the superior mesenteric artery, ventral to the aorta, and ventral to the left renal vein.[13]

17. HEMOBILIA: correct answer e

Hemobilia, or bleeding within the biliary tract, can be treated surgically or nonsurgically. The initial approach for patients with hemobilia is adequate evaluation and resuscitation (including blood transfusions and correction of coagulopathy if necessary), followed by radiologic studies, which include ultrasonography, computed tomography of the abdomen, a red blood cell scan, and angiography. Angiography is considered the most accurate and helpful test. After the diagnosis has been established, selective embolization should be attempted. With hemoperitoneum, management of acute bleeding should be surgical. Direct ligation of vessels, resection, and packing are some of the alternatives for acute hepatic bleeding. Cholecystectomy is the treatment of choice when the bleeding is coming from the gallbladder. A pseudoaneurysm within the liver parenchyma is best treated with embolization or balloon tamponade.

Gastrointestinal bleeding (hematemesis or melena), abdominal pain, and jaundice is the classic triad of hemobilia. This triad occurs in only a minority of patients, and GI bleeding is most common in cases of severe bleeding.

The most common cause of hemobilia is trauma, including surgical procedures, radiologic studies, and extracorporeal lithotripsy. Infections (*Clonorchis* and *Ascaris*) and tumors are two other important causes of hemobilia. Hepatoma is the most common malignant tumor to cause hemobilia.[13]

Quick Answers

1. C	7. C	13. B
2. A	8. E	14. A
3. D	9. D	15. A
4. A	10. D	16. B
5. B	11. A	17. E
6. C	12. A	

REFERENCES

1. Cosenza C, Saffari B, Jabbour N, et al: Surgical management of biliary gallstone disease during pregnancy. Am J Surg 176:545–548, 1999.
2. Graham G, Baxi L, Tharakan T: Laparoscopic cholecystectomy during pregnancy: A case series and review of the literature. Obstet Gynecol Surv 53:566–574, 1998.
3. Sabiston D: The Biological Basis of Modern Surgical Practice, 15th ed. Philadelphia: WB Saunders, 1997, p 281.
4. Sabiston D: The Biological Basis of Modern Surgical Practice, 15th ed. Philadelphia: WB Saunders, 1997, p 848.
5. Valsdottir EB, Isaksson MJ, Kolbeinsson ME: Giant gastric gastrointestinal stromal tumor. Surg Rounds 23:713–715, 2000.
6. Palazzo L, Landi B, Cellier C, et al: Endosonographic features predictive of benign and malignant gastrointestinal stromal cell tumors. Gut 46:88–92, 2000.
7. Nyhus L, Baker R, Fischer J: Mastery of Surgery, 3rd ed. Boston: Little, Brown, 1997, p 546.
8. Sabiston D: The Biological Basis of Modern Surgical Practice, 15th ed. Philadelphia: WB Saunders, 1997, p 1179.

9. Sabiston D: The Biological Basis of Modern Surgical Practice, 15th ed. Philadelphia: WB Saunders, 1997, p 503.
10. Sabiston D: The Biological Basis of Modern Surgical Practice, 15th ed. Philadelphia: WB Saunders, 1997.
11. Cameron JL: Current Surgical Therapy, 6th ed. St Louis: CV Mosby, 1998.
12. Wilson JD, Foster DW, Kronenberg HM, et al: Williams Textbook of Endocrinology, 9th ed. Philadelphia: WB Saunders, 1998.
13. Townsend CM, Sabiston DC, eds: Sabiston Textbook of Surgery: The Biological Basis of Modern Surgical Practice, 16th ed. Philadelphia: WB Saunders, 2001.
14. Feldman M, Scharschmidt BF, Sleisenger MH, et al: Sleisenger & Fordtran's Gastrointestinal and Liver Disease, 6th ed. Philadelphia: WB Saunders, 1998.
15. Evans S, Jackson PG, Czerniach DR, et al: A step-wise approach to laparoscopic Nissen fundoplication: Avoiding technical pitfalls. Arch Surg 135:723–728, 2000.
16. Hunter JG, Smith CD, Branum GD, et al: Laparoscopic fundoplication failures: patterns of failure and response to fundoplication revision. Ann Surg 230:595–604, 1999.
17. Huerta S: Duodenal diverticular disease. Surg Rounds 24:114–127, 2001.
18. Schwartz SI: Principles of Surgery, 7th ed. New York: McGraw-Hill, 1999.
19. Gazelle GS, Saini S, Muller PR: Hepatobiliary and Pancreatic Radiology: Imaging and Intervention. New York: Thieme Medical, 1998.
20. Trotter JF: Liver tumors. Clin Liver Dis 5:17–42, 2001.
21. Feig BW, Berger DH, Fuhrman GM: The M.D. Anderson Surgical Oncology Handbook, 2nd ed. Philadelphia: Lippincott Williams & Wilkins, 1999.
22. Skandalakis JE, Skandalakis PN, Skandalakis LJ: Surgical Anatomy and Technique, A Pocket Manual, 2nd ed. New York: Springer, 1999.
23. O'Leary JP: The Physiologic Basis of Surgery, 2nd ed. Baltimore: Williams & Wilkins, 1996.

NOTES

Lower Gastrointestinal Tract (Small Bowel, Colorectum, and Anus)

QUESTIONS

1. All of the following is true regarding carcinoid tumors except:
   a. Carcinoid heart disease occurs in two thirds of patients with the carcinoid syndrome.
   b. Up to 75% of gastric carcinoid tumors are associated with chronic atrophic gastritis type A.
   c. The majority of patients with small bowel carcinoids present with metastases to the lymph nodes or the liver.
   d. Carcinoid tumors are the second most common cancers of the appendix, and the majority present with signs of obstruction.
   e. Surgical resection of liver metastases may be of benefit (long-term relief of symptoms and prolonged survival) in patients with limited hepatic disease.
2. An otherwise healthy 65-year-old white man presents to your clinic with rectal bleeding. Colonoscopy revealed a 2-cm sessile mass 5 cm from the anal margin. Biopsies were taken that showed a moderate differentiated cancer in situ. What is the most appropriate treatment?
   a. Transanal excision
   b. Low anterior resection

c. Abdominoperineal resection
d. Radiation and chemotherapy only
e. Radiation and chemotherapy, followed by low anterior resection

3. Concerning anal canal cancers, which statement is true?
   a. There is no association between anal cancer and infectious diseases.
   b. The most frequent cancer in this area is adenocarcinoma.
   c. The initial treatment is chemoradiation with complete remission in 70% of cases.
   d. Abdominoperineal resection is always performed after chemoradiation.
   e. Paget disease is an intraepithelial adenocarcinoma that occurs in the elderly and is considered a precancerous lesion.

4. A 65-year-old man comes into your office complaining of melena. He has noticed dark blood per rectum for the past 2 months. He denies any other medical problems. Colonoscopy reveals a mass on the left colon at the level of the splenic flexure. Biopsies show a well-differentiated colon adenocarcinoma. Further work-up for metastatic disease is negative. The patient then undergoes left colectomy without any complications. The specimen reveals a well-differentiated adenocarcinoma invading the muscularis. Two nodes show metastatic disease. What is the cancer staging and the appropriate treatment for this patient?
   a. Dukes C; no further treatment
   b. Dukes B; radiation and chemotherapy
   c. Dukes D; radiation and chemotherapy
   d. Dukes C; chemotherapy
   e. Dukes C; radiation and chemotherapy

5. Six months earlier, a 65-year-old white man underwent a low anterior resection for a rectal cancer that was 7 cm from the anal margin. He comes into your office complaining of rectal bleeding. Colonoscopy shows a biopsy-proven recurrent tumor at the level of the anastomotic suture line. The most appropriate treatment for this patient is:
   a. Chemotherapy alone
   b. Radiation alone
   c. Radiation plus chemotherapy
   d. Abdominoperineal resection
   e. Segmental resection with colostomy

6. Regarding Crohn disease, which one of the following statements is correct?
   a. Initial presentation as an acute abdomen occurs in approximately 35% of patients.
   b. Most cases involve small bowel alone.
   c. Maintenance therapy with steroids is an effective treatment in many patients.
   d. Bypass surgery of diseased bowel is no longer used routinely.
   e. Colonic cancer is not associated with Crohn disease.

7. Regarding colon polyps, which one of the following statements is correct?
   a. Patients with Peutz-Jeghers syndrome should not undergo polyp removal.
   b. Total colectomy with rectal sparing is the surgical treatment of choice for patients with familial adenomatous polyposis.
   c. Gardner syndrome is an autosomic recessive disease.
   d. Patients with Turcot syndrome usually die of colon cancer.

e. Cronkhite-Canada syndrome is associated with villous adenomas.

8. Regarding cecal volvulus, which of the following statements is incorrect?
   a. It is the second most common type of large bowel volvulus.
   b. Patients usually present with small bowel obstruction.
   c. The initial treatment is endoscopic decompression.
   d. The recurrence rate is 20%.
   e. Cecopexy is the most appropriate treatment for cecal volvulus in most patients.

ANSWERS

1. CARCINOID TUMORS: correct answer d

Carcinoid tumors are thought to arise from neuroendocrine cells. In addition to serotonin, carcinoid tumors have been found to secrete corticotropin, histamine, dopamine, substance P, neurotensin, prostaglandins, and kallikrein. The overall incidence of carcinoid tumors in the United States has been estimated to be 1 to 2 cases per 100,000 individuals. The appendix is the most common site of carcinoid tumors, followed by the rectum, ileum, lungs and bronchi, and stomach. Gastric carcinoid tumors make up less than 1% of gastric neoplasms. These tumors can be separated into three distinct groups on the basis of both clinical and histologic characteristics: those associated with chronic atrophic gastritis type A (approximately 75%), those associated with the Zollinger-Ellison syndrome, and sporadic gastric carcinoid tumors. Small bowel carcinoid tumors make up approximately one third of small bowel tumors in surgical series. The majority of patients with small bowel carcinoids presents with metastases to the lymph nodes or the liver, and 5% to 7% present with the carcinoid syndrome. Tumor size is an unreliable predictor of metastatic disease, and metastases have been reported even from tumors measuring less than 0.5 cm in diameter. Long-term survival correlates closely with the stage of the disease at presentation.

Small bowel resection, together with resection of the associated mesentery, is the treatment of choice for small bowel carcinoids. Carcinoid tumors are the most common cancers of the appendix. The size of the tumor is the best predictor of prognosis in patients with appendiceal carcinoid tumors. More than 95% of appendiceal carcinoids are less than 2 cm in diameter. Although metastases from tumors of this size have been reported, they are rare and are usually diagnosed at the time of presentation. In contrast, approximately one third of patients with tumors more than 2 cm in diameter have either nodal or distant metastases. The optimal surgical approach to appendiceal carcinoid tumors has been inferred retrospectively from surgical series. Patients with tumors less than 2 cm in diameter are usually treated by simple appendectomy if there is no gross evidence of local spread. Most tumors more than 2 cm in diameter are treated with right colectomy, since local recurrence following simple appendectomy, although uncommon, has been observed. Whether right colectomy decreases the probability of distant recurrence is unclear. In older patients with other illnesses, simple appendectomy may sometimes be appropriate, even for large tumors. Rectal carcinoid tumors make up 1% to 2% of all rectal tumors and are most common in the sixth decade of life. The size of the primary lesion correlates closely with the probability of metastases, which occur in less than 5% of patients with tumors measuring less than 1 cm in diameter but in the majority of cases in which lesions are more than 2 cm in diameter. Tumors less than 1 cm in diameter account for two thirds of rectal carcinoid tumors and are successfully treated with local excision.

The management of tumors measuring 1 to 2 cm is controversial. Although most tumors of this size can be treated by local excision, several authors have suggested that muscular invasion, symptoms at diagnosis, and ulceration are poor prognostic factors that warrant more extensive surgical procedures. Tumors more than 2 cm in diameter have traditionally been treated by low anterior resection or abdominoperineal resection. The value of these procedures in the treatment of rectal carcinoids has been questioned, however, because such procedures do not appear to extend survival beyond that observed with local excision in retrospective series. An individualized approach, taking into account the patient's age and coexisting conditions, may therefore be appropriate in deciding on a surgical approach to large rectal carcinoids. Patients in whom metastatic disease is suspected should be evaluated with abdominal computed tomography to rule out liver metastases. Liver function tests are an unreliable indicator of tumor involvement of the liver, and the serum alkaline phosphatase level is frequently normal despite extensive involvement of the liver by carcinoid tumor. Measurement of the serotonin metabolite 5-hydroxy-3-indole acetic acid in a 24-hour urine collection may be useful in confirming the diagnosis and in the subsequent monitoring of patients with metastatic carcinoid tumors. Somatostatin analogs have a central role in both the diagnosis and treatment of metastatic carcinoid tumors. Somatostatin is a 14–amino acid peptide that inhibits the secretion of a broad range of hormones, including growth hormone, insulin, glucagon, and gastrin. It acts by binding to somatostatin receptors, which are expressed on more than 80% of carcinoid tumors. Carcinoid heart disease occurs in two thirds of patients with the carcinoid syndrome. Carcinoid heart lesions are characterized by plaque-like, fibrous endocardial thickening that classically involves the right side of the heart and often causes retraction and fixation of the leaflets of the tricuspid and pulmonary valves. Tricuspid regurgitation is a nearly universal finding; tricuspid stenosis, pulmonary regurgitation, and pulmonary stenosis may also occur. Left-sided heart disease occurs in less than 10% of patients. Surgical resection of liver metastases may be of benefit in patients with limited hepatic disease. Such surgery has resulted in long-term relief of symptoms and prolonged survival in selected patients.[1]

2. RECTAL CANCER: correct answer a

Rectal carcinomas that are well or moderately differentiated, located within 10 cm of the anal verge, and less than 3 cm, should be resected by transanal excision. These T1, N0, M0 lesions carry a good prognosis, presenting lymph node metastases in 3% to 10% of cases and conferring a survival rate of more than 90% in 5 years.

Endorectal radiation is another alternative for patients who are not candidates for surgery. One of the disadvantages of this procedure is the absence of a pathologic specimen. Lesions located 10 cm or higher are best managed with a low anterior resection of the rectum.[2–4]

3. ANAL CANCERS: correct answer e

Anal cancers are more frequent in homosexual men, HIV-infected or immunosuppressed persons, and patients with a history of human papilloma virus, herpes simplex virus type I, *Chlamydia trachomatis* infection, and gonorrhea. Anal cancer is more prevalent in patients practicing anal sex, those with poor personal hygiene, and smokers.

The most common histologic type is squamous cell carcinoma, accounting for approximately 80% of the cancers in this area.

Until the 1980s, treatment was based on surgical resection. The prognosis was poor, with low survival rates as a result of distant failure.

Studies showed that chemoradiation is the most effective treatment. The protocol consists of 5-fluorouracil and mitomycin C infusions and radiation therapy (Table 7–1).[5]

Complete remission can be expected in 90% of patients, with a 5-year survival rate of 85%. Abdominoperineal resection is reserved for recurrent disease.

Paget disease is an intraepithelial adenocarcinoma with a well-demarcated eczematoid plaque. Excision with minimal clear margins is the treatment

TABLE 7–1

Chemoradiation for Anal Cancer

Days 1–4	5-Fu, 750–1000 mg/m^2 over 24 hr
Days 1–4	Mitomycin-C, 10–15 mg/m^2, IV bolus
Days 1–35	Radiation therapy 5 days/week for a 45–55 Gy
Days 29–32	5-Fu, 750–1000 mg/m^2 over 24 hr IV

of choice. Paget disease is considered a precancerous lesion.

Bowen disease is an intraepithelial squamous cell cancer, with an irregular plaquelike, eczematoid lesion. Excision is the treatment of choice.[2, 6]

4. COLON CANCER: correct answer d

The original Dukes classification proposed in 1932 was as follows:

A: Lesions confined to the bowel wall
B: Lesions through the bowel wall, but with no involvement of nodes
C: Lesions with lymph node involvement

Dukes classification was later modified as follows:

A: Lesions confined to mucosa and submucosa
B1: Lesions extending to but not through muscularis propria
B2: Lesions extending through muscularis propria into pericolonic fat
C1: Lesions limited to the bowel wall, with positive lymph nodes
C2: Lesions invading all layers, with positive lymph nodes

It is not uncommon to stage tumors with distant metastasis as Dukes D, although it was not part of the original classification.

Fifty percent to 60% of patients with colon cancer have tumors that penetrate the serosa or involve the regional nodes. This group of patients will benefit from adjuvant chemotherapy with 5-fluorouracil and levamisole, reducing by 41% the chances of recurrence and decreasing the overall mortality rate by 33%. Radiation therapy has not been shown to be effective in colon cancer as it has in patients with rectal cancer.[7]

5. COLORECTAL CANCER: correct answer d

Recurrent colon cancer occurs in almost half of patients who undergo curative primary resection. Undetectable malignancy at the time of the primary operation is the most common cause of recurrence. Many options are available for the treatment of colorectal cancer, including radiation, chemotherapy, and surgery. Surgical resection remains the modality with the best potential for cure. Whenever possible, surgery should be considered.

Since recurrence usually occurs in the first 3 years after resection, patients should undergo surveillance, which will include a carcinoembryonic antigen level determination every 6 to 8 weeks, computed tomography of the abdomen and pelvis every 6 months, and annual colonoscopy.[7, 8]

6. CROHN DISEASE: correct answer d

Only 10% of patients with Crohn disease present initially with a clinical picture similar to appendicitis. Most patients have intermittent pain and diarrhea, which usually does not contain mucus, pus, or blood. About 50% of cases involve the small bowel and large bowel. In 30% of patients, only the small bowel is involved, and in the remaining 20% the colon alone is diseased. Steroids should be used only in the acute setting, not as maintenance therapy. Steroids do not cure or prevent recurrence of the disease and add significant morbidity when used chronically because of their many side effects.

Bypass of the diseased segment is rarely used today. The bypass bowel segment that is affected by Crohn disease will be an active source of the disease and cause complications.

Ulcerative colitis and Crohn disease are associated with colon cancer, although the incidence of colon tumor is much higher in patients with ulcerative colitis.[7, 8]

7. COLON POLYPS: correct answer b

Hyperplastic polyps are not considered malignant or premalignant lesions. Conversely, *adenomatous polyps*, which include *tubular*, *villous*, and *tubulovillous polyps*, are considered premalignant lesions. Villous adenomas occur most frequently in the sigmoid and rectum and have the greatest potential among adenomatous polyps to become malignant.

Familial adenomatous polyposis is an autosomal dominant disease, with almost 100% penetrance, which presents with hundreds of thousands of colonic polyps that are premalignant. Most patients who not undergo resection of the colon by age 40 experience colon cancer. Several surgical options are available, including total proctocolectomy with continent ileostomy (Koch pouch), total proctocolectomy with ileal pouch anal anastomosis, or total colectomy with ileorectal anastomosis, in which the patient will have to undergo frequent endoscopic surveillance of the rectal stump.

Gardner syndrome is an autosomal dominant disease characterized by multiple polyps on the colon, stomach, and small bowel and the presence of desmoid tumors, supernumerary teeth, and mandibular cysts.

Turcot syndrome is an autosomal recessive disease characterized by multiple adenomas of the colon and the presence of central nervous system tumors. Patients usually die of the central nervous system disease and not of colon cancer.

Peutz-Jeghers syndrome is an autosomal dominant disease characterized by multiple hamartomas of the stomach, small bowel, and colon; mucocutaneous pigmentation; nasal and bronchial polyps; and, rarely, ovarian cysts and bladder polyps. These patients are at increased risk for mainly small bowel cancer because of associated adenomatous polyps. Because of this, whenever diagnosed, polyps should be removed endoscopically.[7]

8. CECAL VOLVULUS: correct answer c

Unlike sigmoid volvulus, endoscopic decompression is not indicated for cecal volvulus. Patients with cecal volvulus must undergo exploratory laparotomy. The first thing to be done in the operating theater is to reduce the volvulus and check bowel viability. If viability is questionable, bowel resection should be performed, followed by an ileostomy and mucous fistula or primary anastomosis to the transverse colon.

Most patients have viable colon. In these patients, volvulus detorsion and cecopexy alone is the most appropriate treatment.

Recurrence alone occurs in about 20% of cases, so detorsion alone is not an adequate treatment.

All patients with cecal volvulus eventually need evaluation of the distal large bowel to check for any lesions that may have led to cecal distention.[2, 7]

Quick Answers

1. D	4. D	7. B
2. A	5. D	8. C
3. E	6. D	

REFERENCES

1. Kulke M, Mayers R: Medical progress: carcinoid tumors. N Engl J Med 11:858–868, 1999.
2. Cameron JL: Current Surgical Therapy, 6th ed. St. Louis: CV Mosby, 1998.
3. Abeloff MD: Clinical Oncology, 2nd ed. New York: Churchill Livingstone, 2000.
4. Feldman N, Scharschmidt BF, Sleisenger MH, Klein S: Sleisenger & Fordtran's Gastrointestinal and Liver Disease, 6th ed. Philadelphia: WB Saunders, 1998.
5. Feig BW, Berger DM, Fuhrman GM: The MD Anderson Surgical Oncology Handbook, 2nd ed. Philadelphia: Lippincott Williams & Wilkins, 1999.
6. Nigro ND: Multidisciplinary management of cancer of the anus. World T Surg 11:446–451, 1987.
7. Townsend CM, Sabiston DC, eds: Sabiston Textbook of Surgery: The Biological Basis of Modern Surgical Practice, 16th ed. Philadelphia: WB Saunders, 2001.
8. McQuarrie DG, Humphrey EW, Lee JT: Reoperative General Surgery, 2nd ed. St. Louis: CV Mosby, 1998.

NOTES

Breast

QUESTIONS

1. A 52-year-old white woman with a positive family history of breast cancer (four maternal aunts affected before age 40) undergoes genetic testing. The testing demonstrates that she is a *BRCA1* carrier, and she returns for further recommendations. She is postmenopausal and receiving hormone replacement therapy with an unremarkable physical examination. All of the following are appropriate recommendations except:
   a. Prophylactic oophorectomy and annual breast cancer screening
   b. Option of bilateral mastectomy
   c. Option of chemoprevention with tamoxifen
   d. Discontinuance of hormone replacement therapy
   e. Annual breast and ovarian cancer screening

2. Two weeks after a modified radical mastectomy for breast cancer, a 56-year-old woman returns to your clinic with the winged scapula deformity. Which nerve was injured during the procedure?
   a. Subscapular nerve
   b. Long thoracic nerve
   c. Thoracodorsal nerve
   d. Intercostal brachial nerve
   e. Suprascapular nerve

3. All of the following are contraindications to breast conservation surgery therapy except:
   a. Multicentricity
   b. Pregnancy (first and second trimesters)

c. Lupus
d. Follow-up not possible
e. Tumor adherent to the chest wall

4. A 52-year-old white woman comes to your office after 1 week of vacationing in Florida. Her major complaint is sunburn on her left breast. Physical examination reveals a sunburned face and an erythematous, warm-to-the-touch left breast. Breast biopsy reveals inflammatory breast cancer. The best approach and treatment for this patient is:
   a. Chemotherapy and radiation therapy
   b. Modified radical mastectomy
   c. Partial mastectomy followed by radiation therapy
   d. Chemotherapy only
   e. Chemotherapy, followed by modified radical mastectomy and radiation therapy

5. Which of the following treatments for different breast conditions is correct?
   a. The treatment for cystosarcoma phyllodes is total (simple) mastectomy with axillary lymph node dissection.
   b. The treatment for lobular carcinoma in situ is total mastectomy without axillary node dissection.
   c. The treatment for intraductal carcinoma in situ is total mastectomy without axillary node dissection.
   d. The treatment for isolated Paget disease of the breast is mastectomy with axillary node dissection.
   e. The treatment for intraductal papilloma of the breast is simple mastectomy.

6. What is the percentage of breast microcalcifications that will turn out to be malignant?
   a. 5%

b. 15%
c. 30%
d. 50%
e. 80%

7. Stewart-Treves syndrome is characterized by:
   a. Skin angiosarcoma due to persistent edematous upper extremity after a mastectomy
   b. Angiosarcoma of the breast after radiation therapy
   c. Multiple sarcomas and carcinomas, including breast cancer
   d. Multiple hamartomas associated with breast cancer
   e. Involvement of the breast skin epidermis with clear abundant cytoplasm and pleomorphic nuclei cells causing a black discoloration after chemotherapy

8. A 35-year-old white woman comes into your office complaining of right breast tenderness and thickening of her right breast tissue. She does not have any other medical problems. On physical examination, her right breast is somewhat tender on the right upper quadrant with dense breast tissue at palpation. A mammogram shows microcalcifications on the right upper quadrant. Needle local biopsy is performed, which reveals atypical epithelial hyperplasia associated with cysts lined by large polygonal cells having an abundant granular, eosinophilic cytoplasm with small, round, deeply chromatic nuclei. What is the most appropriate treatment for this patient?
   a. Simple mastectomy
   b. Modified radical mastectomy
   c. Lumpectomy and radiation
   d. Lumpectomy and sentinel lymph node biopsy
   e. Close observation

9. Regarding breast cancer recurrence, which one of the following statements is true?
   a. Axillary nodes constitute the most frequent site of local recurrence.
   b. Most patients with local recurrence have concomitant metastatic disease.
   c. The median survival time after recurrence of breast cancer is 10 years.
   d. Radiation therapy plays a minimal role in breast cancer recurrence.
   e. The recurrence rate of breast tumor after lumpectomy and radiation is 8% in 8 years.

10. A 55-year-old black woman comes into your office complaining of a palpable lump on her right breast. She states that her mother and aunt had breast cancer. She has no other medical problems. On physical examination, you notice a palpable mass of 4 cm on the outer quadrant of her right breast. There are no palpable axillary nodes. Fine-needle aspiration reveals ductal infiltrating carcinoma. What is the preoperative clinical stage for this patient?
    a. IB
    b. IIA
    c. IIB
    d. IIIA
    e. IV

ANSWERS

1. BREAST-OVARIAN CANCER SYNDROME: correct answer e

Familial breast cancer accounts for 5% to 10% of all breast cancers, and a substantial number of these cases can be linked to mutations in the genes *BRCA1* or *BRCA2*. Familial cases of ovarian cancer account for up to 8% of all ovarian cancers, and recent reports suggest that most if not all of these cases may be traced to mutations in *BRCA1* or *BRCA2*. The transmission follows an autosomal dominant pattern. It is estimated that carriers have a 50% to 85% chance of developing breast cancer by the age of 70 and a 16% to 60% risk of ovarian cancer. In addition, *BRCA1* mutation carriers are also found to have a higher incidence of prostate and colon cancer, whereas *BRCA2* families appear to have an increased incidence of male breast cancer. *BRCA1* is linked to chromosome 17 and *BRCA2* is linked to chromosome 13. *BRCA1*-associated tumors are more likely to be aneuploid, have a high S-phase component, be high-grade, and be negative for estrogen and progesterone receptors. Some estimates are that 1 of every 200 women in the United States harbors a germline mutation in *BRCA1.* Moreover, women of Ashkenazi Jewish heritage in the United States have a higher incidence of germline mutations in *BRCA1* (3 to 4 per 100 women).[1]

For those who desire genetic testing, adequate genetic counseling is required before and after the acquisition of any testing results. Those with positive results have many treatment options, including various screening methods, chemoprevention, and prophylactic surgery. Unlike breast cancer, ovarian cancer screening has not been shown to be effective, and prophylactic bilateral oophorectomy is the procedure of choice. However, because the risk of ovarian cancer increases in the late 40s and early 50s, women may wait until after childbearing is complete before choosing to undergo surgery.[2]

2. BREAST ANATOMY: correct answer b

Coursing close to the chest wall on the medial side of the axilla is the long thoracic nerve, or the external respiratory nerve of Bell, which innervates the serratus anterior muscle. This muscle is important in fixation of the scapula to the chest wall during adduction of the shoulder and extension of the arm, and its denervation results in the winged scapula deformity. For this reason, the long thoracic nerve is carefully preserved during standard axillary dissection. The thoracodorsal nerve innervates the latissimus dorsi muscle.[3]

3. BREAST CANCER: correct answer e

In patients with stage I and stage II breast cancer, lumpectomy with axillary node dissection and irradiation or modified radical mastectomy are alternative treatments.

The choice of breast conservative treatment should be made carefully, following the basic principles of breast conservation surgery. The surgeon should be able to resect the tumor without compromise of the breast architecture. Patients with multiple tumors usually have heavily microscopic tumor burdens throughout the breast, leading to high local failure rates.

Radiation cannot be safely delivered during the first and second trimesters of pregnancy. For patients in the last trimester, lumpectomy plus axillary node dissection plus radiation is an option.

Reports have shown that patients with lupus and scleroderma experience breast necrosis and fibrosis after radiation treatment. Radiation should be avoided in these patients.

The failure rate of breast conservative treatment is approximately 8% to 10%. Follow-up in all patients is essential to "catch" the recurrent cases.

Depth of the tumor, histologic type or grade, patient age, and family history are not contraindications for conservative breast cancer treatment.[4, 5]

4. INFLAMMATORY BREAST CANCER: correct answer e

Inflammatory breast cancer was named by Lee and Tannenbaum in 1924 but had been described earlier in the century. The breast is erythematous, edematous, and warm and tender to the touch, with a palpable tumor in 70% of cases. Palpable nodes are found in 50% to 60% of cases. The differential diagnosis includes breast bacterial infections, postradiation dermatitis, sarcoma, leukemia, and lymphoma.

When inflammatory breast cancer is suspected, a bilateral mammogram should be obtained. Tissue biopsy should be performed to confirm the clinical impression. Skin biopsy results show dermal lymphatic invasion. The initial treatment consists of multimodality chemotherapy with 5-fluorouracil, doxorubicin, cyclophosphamide, vincristine, and prednisone followed by a modified radical mastectomy and irradiation.

Clinical response to initial chemotherapy is highly predictive of a good outcome. Patients with complete or partial response to induction chemotherapy experience improved disease-specific and disease-free survival.[4, 6, 7]

5. BREAST DISEASE: correct answer c

Intraductal carcinoma in situ of the breast can be treated with total mastectomy or by lumpectomy, followed by breast irradiation. The recurrence rate of the former treatment is approximately 2%, and the recurrence rate with the latter treatment is 8%. No axillary node dissection is necessary because of the low rate of metastasis to the axilla (<2%) in intraductal carcinoma in situ of the breast.

Patients with cystosarcoma phyllodes should undergo resection of the lesion or a simple mastectomy if the tumor has invaded the adjacent tissue locally.

Lobular carcinoma in situ of the breast is considered a tumor marker and is usually an incidental finding after a breast biopsy. Bilateral prophylactic total mastectomy or close follow-up can be recommended.

Paget disease of the breast presents with redness, itching, and thickening of the nipple-areola complex. A simple mastectomy is the treatment of choice. If invasive breast cancer is found concomitant with Paget disease, an axillary node dissection should be performed.

Papillomas of the breast are the most common tumors to present with bloody nipple discharge. If no other masses are present, the treatment of choice is ductal excision through a subareolar wedge resection.[4, 5, 8]

6. BREAST CANCER: correct answer b

About 15% of microcalcifications are associated with malignant disease. Clustered calcifications, smaller than 0.5 mm, are more commonly associated with malignancy than are larger, coarse calcifications. Biopsy of these lesions is mandatory. Ductal carcinoma in situ frequently presents as an area of microcalcification.[9]

7. BREAST CANCER: correct answer a

Stewart-Treves syndrome is characterized by skin angiosarcoma of a persistent edematous arm after a mastectomy. Angiosarcoma of the breast is most likely associated with radiation therapy. There is a 0.3% to 0.4% risk of angiosarcoma after radiation therapy of the breast, with most cases arising after 5 to 10 years of treatment.

Women with Cowden disease ("multiple hamartoma syndrome," due to a mutation of a gene on chromosome 10q) have a 30% to 50% risk of breast cancer by age 50.

Li-Fraumeni syndrome is characterized by multiple sarcomas and carcinomas, including breast cancer. Early-onset breast cancer occurs along with soft tissue sarcomas, osteosarcoma, leukemia, brain tumors, adrenal cortical tumors, and other cancers.

Paget disease is characterized by cells with abundant clear cytoplasm and pleomorphic nuclei involving the epidermis of the breast. Patients present with erythema, edema, and ulceration of the nipple-areola complex.[7, 9, 10]

8. BREAST: correct answer e

Patients with atypical epithelial hyperplasia (a tumor marker) may experience breast cancer later in life. Close follow-up and advice are indicated. No surgical intervention is necessary.

Fibrocystic changes of the breast are common in young patients. Patients usually complain of breast pain and thickening of the breast tissue. No surgical treatment is necessary for fibrocystic disease.[7, 9]

9. BREAST CANCER: correct answer e

Breast cancer recurs in about 8% of patients after 8 years of breast conservation therapy and irradiation, and in 2% of patients 10 years after radical mastectomy for breast cancer stages I to II.

The median survival rate after recurrence is only 3 years, and the tumor recurs at least half of the time on the chest wall. Recurrence to the axillary nodes alone occurs in approximately 10% of these patients. In 20% to 30% of patients, metastatic disease is present when local recurrence has been diagnosed.

Reoperation, radiation therapy, and chemotherapy are important in the treatment of recurrent disease.[11]

10. BREAST CANCER AND TNM STAGING: correct answer b

TNM staging is used as guide for treatment and as a prognostic indicator for breast cancer.

T is for tumor size and is used for carcinoma in situ: intraductal carcinoma, lobular carcinoma in situ, or Paget disease of the nipple with no tumor. T1, tumor <2 cm; T2, tumor between 2 and 5 cm; T3, tumor >5 cm; T4, chest wall or direct skin involvement.

N is used for lymph nodes: N1, suspicious mobile axillary nodes; N2, fixed axillary nodes; N3, ipsilateral internal mammary nodes.

M is used for metastasis: M0, no metastasis; M1, involvement of supraclavicular nodes, liver, bone, or lungs.

Table 8–1 describes the stage grouping according to the American Joint Committee on Cancer and the International Union Against Cancer (AJCC/UICC).

Quick Answers

1. E	6. B
2. B	7. A
3. E	8. E
4. E	9. E
5. C	10. B

TABLE 8–1

AJCC Breast Cancer Staging

Stage Grouping			
Stage 0	Tis	N0	M0
Stage I	T1*	N0	M0
Stage IIA	T0	N1	M0
	T1*	N1**	M0
	T2	N0	M0
Stage IIB	T2	N1	M0
	T3	N0	M0
Stage IIIA	T0	N2	M0
	T1*	N2	M0
	T2	N2	M0
	T3	N1	M0
	T3	N2	M0
Stage IIIB	T4	Any N	M0
	Any T	N3	M0
Stage IV	Any T	Any N	M1

*Note : T1 includes T1 mic
**Note : The prognosis of patients with N1a is similar to the patients with pN0.
+From American Joint Committee on Cancer: AJCC Cancer Staging Handbook, 5th ed. Philadelphia: Lippincott-Raven, 1998.

REFERENCES

1. Holland J, Frei E: Cancer Medicine, 5th ed. Hamilton: American Cancer Society, 2000, pp 168–169.
2. Bitran J: Expert Guide to Oncology, 1st ed. Philadelphia: American College of Physicians, 2000, pp 15–19.

3. Sabiston D: The Biological Basis of Modern Surgical Practice, 15th ed. Philadelphia: WB Saunders, 1997, p 556.
4. Cameron JL: Current Surgical Therapy, 6th ed. St Louis: CV Mosby, 1998.
5. Fisher B: Eight-year results of a randomized clinical trial comparing total mastectomy and lumpectomy with or without irradiation in the treatment of breast cancer. N Engl J Med 320:822–828, 1989.
6. Lopez MJ, Porter KA: Inflammatory breast cancer. Surg Clin North Am 76:411–429, 1996.
7. Cotran RS: Robbins Pathologic Basis of Disease, 6th ed. Philadelphia: WB Saunders, 1999.
8. Fisher B, Constantino J, Redmond C, et al: Lumpectomy compared with lumpectomy with radiation therapy for the treatment of intraductal breast cancer. N Engl J Med 328:1581–1586, 1993.
9. Townsend CM, Sabiston DC, eds: Sabiston Textbook of Surgery: The Biological Basis of Modern Surgical Practice, 16th ed. Philadelphia: WB Saunders, 2001.
10. Abeloff MD: Clinical Oncology, 2nd ed. New York: Churchill Livingstone, 2000.
11. McQuarrie DG, Humphrey EW, Lee JT: Reoperative general surgery, 2nd ed. St. Louis: CV Mosby, 1998.

NOTES

Trauma and Critical Care

QUESTIONS

1. A 65-year-old woman with a history of coronary artery disease (three myocardial infarctions, including one that occurred 2 months earlier), chronic renal disease (which had resulted in the patient's dependence on dialysis for 4 years), insulin-dependent diabetes, and peripheral vascular disease presented with a cold, painful left foot requiring revascularization. The surgeon, the anesthesiology team, and the cardiology consultant agreed that the patient probably would not tolerate cross-clamping of her aorta, which would have been needed to bypass her stenotic left iliac (the lesion was not amenable to stenting). A left axillary-femoral bypass was the next option. The right radial arterial catheter was nonfunctional during several intervals of the case when the proximal subclavian artery was clamped. During one of those clamped periods, the mixed venous oxygen (Svo_2) decreased from 73% to 58% over just a few minutes. All the following can cause a decrease in Svo_2 in such a patient except:
   a. A decline in the cardiac output from the previous measurement of 4.1 to 3.2 L/min
   b. Decreased hematocrit and Spo_2 (pulse oximeter)
   c. A left shift of the oxygen-hemoglobin dissociation curve

d. Changes in the electrocardiogram ST-segment analysis
e. Respiratory distress syndrome (poor vent setting)

2. When performing an emergency open cricothyroidotomy, the skin incision should be made:
   a. Over the cricothyroid membrane
   b. 1 cm cephalad to the cricothyroid membrane
   c. 1 cm caudal to the cricothyroid membrane
   d. Over the upper border of the thyroid cartilage
   e. Over the lower border of the cricoid cartilage

3. After a blunt thoracic trauma, which cardiac structure is most commonly injured?
   a. Right atrium
   b. Right ventricle
   c. Left atrium
   d. Left ventricle
   e. Interventricular septum

4. A 65-year-old white man underwent a total gastrectomy with Roux-en-Y esophagojejunostomy because of gastric carcinoma. After surgery, his feeding tube jejunostomy clogged. Central venous hyperalimentation was needed. A central line was placed at the right subclavian site. After line placement, the patient experienced hypotension and you noticed distended neck veins. The most likely cause is:
   a. Kinking of the superior and inferior venae cavae
   b. Free atrial wall perforation
   c. Obstruction of the right ventricle outlet
   d. Thrombosis of the right heart inflow
   e. Embolism to the pulmonary artery

5. A 30-year-old white male restrained driver involved in a motor vehicle accident presented

to the emergency shock room with hypotension and tachycardia. The chest radiograph revealed widening of the mediastinum. An aortogram was obtained, which showed a thoracic aortic injury. The correct statement considering thoracic aortic injuries is:
   a. The most common location is the ascending aorta.
   b. The operative mortality rate ranges from 10% to 20%.
   c. Posterolateral right thoracotomy allows cross-clamping of the descending aorta and is the surgical approach of choice.
   d. The postoperative incidence of spinal cord injury is approximately 30%.
   e. Most patients complain of chest pain and back pain.

6. During diagnostic peritoneal lavage (closed technique), the needle should be inserted:
   a. In the midline, at one third the distance from the umbilicus to the symphysis pubis
   b. In the midline, at two thirds the distance from the umbilicus to the symphysis pubis
   c. In the midline, at half the distance from the umbilicus to the symphysis pubis
   d. In the midline, 2 cm below the umbilicus
   e. In the center on an imaginary triangle between the umbilicus and the anterior superior iliac spines

7. After a fall, a 77-year-old woman presents to the emergency department with pain, tenderness, and instability of the right arm. Radiographs show a midshaft humerus fracture. The most likely nerve injured in this situation is the
   a. Musculocutaneous nerve
   b. Median nerve

c. Ulnar nerve
d. Radial nerve
e. Medial cutaneous nerve of the arm

8. A 29-year-old white woman with a history of asthma underwent total thyroidectomy because of papillary carcinoma of the thyroid. In the recovery room, she experienced stridor and difficulty breathing. Her oxygen saturation dropped to 85%, and she had perioral and extremity cyanosis. Which of the following is the most appropriate treatment for this patient?
   a. Tracheostomy
   b. Orotracheal intubation
   c. Nonrebreather mask, inhalers, and chest therapy
   d. Nasal intubation
   e. Laryngeal airway mask insertion

9. A 28-year-old man sustained a dog bite to his right arm. His physical examination revealed a large, open wound at his forearm and loss of motor function and sensation at the radial nerve distribution. Exploring the wound at bedside, you notice total transection of the radial nerve. Radiographs showed no fractured bones. What is the most appropriate treatment for this patient?
   a. Exploration of the wound in the operating room with primary repair of the transected nerve
   b. Immediate local wound care, antibiotic administration, and delayed repair of the nerve
   c. Immediate cleansing of the wound, antibiotic administration, and no repair of the nerve
   d. Immediate cleansing of the wound, antibiotic administration, observation for 24 hours, and then exploration and repair in the operating room

e. Exploration of the wound in the operating room, with a transposition muscle flap over the injured nerve

10. A 25-year-old man involved in a car accident is found to have a complete transection of the pancreas at the level of the pancreatic neck. What is the most appropriate surgical treatment for this patient?
    a. Roux-en-Y pancreaticojejunostomy of the proximal pancreas and distal pancreatectomy
    b. Drainage of the proximal and distal segments
    c. Drainage of the proximal segment and oversewing of the distal segment
    d. Oversewing of the proximal segment and drainage of the distal segment
    e. Oversewing of the proximal segment and distal pancreatectomy

11. A 45-year-old man was kicked several times in his abdomen in a bar fight. He came to the emergency department complaining of being unable to void for 24 hours. Insertion of a Foley catheter revealed gross hematuria with clots and persistent hematuria after irrigation. Excretory urography followed by retrograde urethrocystography showed the absence of kidney or urethral injury but the presence of contrast material superior to the bladder into the paracolic gutters. Appropriate treatment includes which of the following?
    a. Urinary catheter drainage (Foley)
    b. Urinary catheter drainage with continuous bladder irrigation
    c. Bilateral nephrostomy tubes
    d. Suprapubic catheter drainage
    e. Exploratory laparotomy with oversewing of the bladder wall

ANSWERS

1. MIXED VENOUS OXYGEN TENSION (Svo_2): correct answer c

An important way of assessing tissue oxygen delivery is to evaluate the mixed venous oxygen level. Svo_2 provides one of the most important assessments of tissue oxygen metabolism; recall that accurate sampling of true Svo_2 requires sampling of the pulmonary artery. The normal Svo_2 is 65% to 75%. The factors that determine Svo_2 are several and include

Cardiac output
Oxygen consumption
Amount of hemoglobin
Loading of hemoglobin
Saturation of hemoglobin

The determinants of Svo_2 are identified by rearranging the Fick equation:

$$Svo_2 = Sao_2 - (Vo_2 \div CO \times Hb \times 1.3)$$

where CO = cardiac output, Hb = hemoglobin, Sao_2 = arterial oxygen saturation, and Vo_2 = consumption of oxygen.

Factors that cause low Svo_2 as you would predict from this equation are increased Vo_2 in hypermetabolic states (such as fever, exercise, agitation, shivering, or thyrotoxicosis); low CO secondary to myocardial infarction, congestive heart failure, or hypovolemia; low Sao_2 from respiratory distress syndrome (poor vent settings); high oxygen consumption; anemia; a right shift of the oxygen-hemoglobin dissociation curve causing increased unloading of hemoglobin at the tissue level (sickle cell disease); hypoxia; or any other factor causing a low hemoglobin saturation. The most common cause of a high Svo_2 is a wedged catheter. Sao_2 is probably not significant unless there has been a prolonged hypoxia. Vo_2 can be low secondary to sepsis, hypothermia, and cases of metabolic poisoning such as cyanide toxicity, carbon monoxide poisoning, and methemoglobinemias (severe left shift of the oxyhemoglobin dissociation curve resulting in decreased unloading of hemoglobin at the tissue level). CO can be high secondary to burns, sepsis, left-to-right shunts, arteriovenous fistulas, hepatitis, and pancreatitis. Hemoglobin cannot significantly raise the Svo_2.[1]

2. EMERGENCY CRICOTHYROIDOTOMY: correct answer a

Emergency cricothyroidotomy is intended to provide emergency access to the airway in patients in whom orotracheal intubation is either technically impossible or unsafe. The surgical technique involves the identification of the cricothyroid membrane between the lower border of the thyroid cartilage and the upper border of the cricoid cartilage. A horizontal (sometimes vertical) incision is made. A No. 11 blade is inserted into the cricothyroid membrane, and the opening in the membrane is extended horizontally. The back of the knife handle or a hemostat is used to open the airway so that a No. 4 or No. 6 Shiley tracheostomy or an endotracheal tube can be inserted.[2]

3. BLUNT CARDIAC INJURY: correct answer b

The right ventricle is most frequently involved because of its proximity to the sternum.

4. CENTRAL VENOUS LINES: correct answer a

Several complications are associated with central line placement. One of the most common is pneumothorax. In this case, the patient experiences a tension pneumothorax, wherein a flap valve allows air to enter the intrapleural space but prevents its escape. Intrapleural pressure rises, the lung collapses, and the mediastinum shifts to the opposite side. Cardiac function is impaired from kinking of the superior and inferior venae cavae. Treatment should be immediate chest needle decompression followed by chest tube thoracostomy.

Catheter erosion through the atrial wall has been reported with catastrophic outcomes. Subclavian thrombosis occurs in 5% to 10% of patients with central lines. Thrombolytic therapy should be started. After streptokinase therapy, heparin should be continued for 1 to 2 weeks and warfarin for 6 months.

Superior vena cava obstruction due to placement of indwelling catheters has become more common. Patients present with edema of the neck, head, and upper extremities; cyanosis; headache; and distended neck veins. The rapid occlusion of the superior vena cava causes cerebral edema and intracranial thrombosis that can lead to coma and death.[4]

Pulmonary embolism is associated with dyspnea, hypoxemia, tachycardia, hypotension, and right ventricle enlargement. It is associated with poor central line placement technique (e.g., the patient was not in the Trendelenburg position or the line was not properly flushed). Several techniques can help in the diagnosis of a pulmonary embolism, including chest radiography (to rule out pneumothorax, pulmonary edema, or adult respiratory distress syndrome), electrocardiography (to rule out pericarditis or myocardial infarction), arterial blood gas determinations, ventilation-perfusion scans, and pulmonary angiography (gold standard).[5, 6]

5. TRAUMATIC AORTIC INJURIES: correct answer b

Traumatic aortic injuries occur frequently. Ninety percent of patients with this injury die at the scene; 40% will die if no surgical intervention is performed. The surgical mortality rate ranges from 10% to 20%.

Patients usually have no complaints. Symptoms and signs that can raise suspicion of an aortic injury include chest and back pain, chest abrasions and bruises, seat belt "tracks" in the chest, decreased lower extremity pulses, and lower extremity neurologic impairment. It is imperative for the surgeon to document neurologic impairment at the initial evaluation because of the 7% incidence of paraplegia after thoracic aortic repair.

The most common site of thoracic aortic injury is at the descending aorta. At the level of the ligamentum arteriosum, the aorta is fixed, being extremely vulnerable to rupture.[7–9]

6. PERITONEAL LAVAGE: correct answer a

After the urinary bladder and the stomach are decompressed, the needle should be inserted in the midline, at one third the distance from the umbilicus to the symphysis pubis.[10]

7. ANATOMY: correct answer d

The radial nerve courses laterally in the arm and may be injured in open fractures or fractures at the junction of the middle and distal thirds of the humerus. At this point, the nerve is close to the humerus. In most instances, the injury is caused by stretching or contusion, and function returns within several weeks to 6 months. In open fractures involving the radial nerve or in fractures with soft tissue interposition, exploration of the radial nerve is indicated. Delayed suturing is acceptable, but the decision depends on the lesion.[11]

8. RECURRENT LARYNGEAL NERVE INJURY: correct answer b

During neck surgery, two nerves play a major role in postoperative complications: the *superior laryngeal nerve* and the *recurrent laryngeal nerve.* The superior laryngeal nerve provides motor and sensory innervations to the larynx and, when injured, causes bowing of the vocal cord during phonation. This injury is noted only in professional singers or speakers who use high-pitched notes. The superior laryngeal nerve is found medial and inferior to the carotid artery and divides into two branches: a sensory internal laryngeal branch and an external motor branch. The internal branch is rarely identified by the surgeon, but the external branch passes under the sternocleidomastoid muscle together with the superior thyroid vein and artery and innervates the cricothyroid muscle.

The recurrent laryngeal nerve is a branch of the vagus nerve and has different pathways before entering the neck. The right recurrent laryngeal nerve crosses the subclavian artery anteriorly, loops around the artery anteroposteriorly, and ascends in the tracheoesophageal groove, passing posterior to the right thyroid lobe to enter the larynx. The left recurrent laryngeal nerve loops around the aorta and ascends in the tracheoesophageal groove to enter the larynx. In less than 1% of patients, the right laryngeal nerve does not loop around the subclavian artery and is called the *nonrecurrent laryngeal nerve*.[5, 12]

During thyroidectomy, the laryngeal nerve should be recognized at the level where it enters the larynx, posterior to the inferior cornu of the thyroid cartilage.

The recurrent laryngeal nerve provides motor innervation to most of the laryngeal muscles. Its unilateral injury leads to a unilateral vocal cord paralysis and hoarseness. Bilateral injury to this nerve severely compromises the airway, and a tracheostomy becomes necessary.[13]

9. PERIPHERAL NERVE TRANSECTION: correct answer b

Peripheral nerve injuries can be classified into five degrees. *First degree* is called *neurapraxia,* involving some conduction loss but no anatomic damage. *Second degree* is called *axonotmesis* and presents as an axonal disruption without loss of the neurolemmal sheath. Full recovery should be expected. *Third-degree* injuries involve loss of the nerve sheaths. In third-degree injuries, when axons are regenerating they may enter the nerve sheaths incorrectly, resulting in aberrant regeneration. The time of recovery depends on the length of the nerve that was injured. The rate of regeneration is about 1 mm/day. In *fourth-degree* injuries, there is fascicular disruption. A great amount of scarring and inflammation is present; therefore, axons have to grow through this intraneural scarring to become functional. Most patients with this degree of injury benefit from nerve repair. *Fifth-degree* injuries involve total nerve transection. All patients require wound exploration and nerve repair. In clean, sharp, totally transected nerves, repair can be done immediately. Delayed repair is preferred by most surgeons for many reasons, especially in dirty, macerated wounds. The delayed repair turns the scenario into a benign and elective case, allows the wound to heal, and decreases the chances of infection. The scarred ends of the nerve are better visualized, and there is a clear-cut edge between injured and noninjured nerve. Delayed repair of a totally transected nerve should not be postponed more than 1 month. Indeed, 3 weeks is when neurons have their maximal level of regenerative activity after injury.

Gunshot wounds, crushing blows, traction, and fractures can be explored by 2 months if signs of recovery are absent. If the injury to the nerve is within 2 to 3 inches of the first recoverable muscle, which at 2 months may be on the verge of reinnervation, an additional delay of 1 more month may be justified. If there is no improvement by 3 months, exploration and repair should be performed.

The brachial plexus is an exception. For stretches or contusions, patients can be observed for 4 months.[14]

10. PANCREATIC TRAUMA: correct answer e

The most frequent injuries to the pancreas after blunt trauma are contusions or capsular lacerations. These injuries require hemostasis and external drainage only. In these injuries, if the drainage output of amylase is less than the concentration in the serum, the drain can be removed 24 to 48 hours after surgery. If the drainage fluid contains a high amylase concentration, the drain should be kept until there is no more evidence of a pancreatic leak.

The pancreatic neck is a common site of injury in blunt trauma. Total pancreatic neck transection is best treated with distal pancreatectomy and oversewing of the proximal stump. The transected pancreatic duct should be directly suture-ligated with nonabsorbable stitches, and the parenchyma oversewn with absorbable or nonabsorbable mattress sutures. If there is concern about the proximal pancreatic duct, pancreatography should be performed. If stenosis of the proximal pancreatic duct is noticed, the open proximal end of the duct can be drained into a Roux-en-Y jejunal limb. If there is concern that the proximal pancreatic parenchyma is inadequate, preservation of the distal pancreatic tail should be attempted, with a Roux-en-Y pancreaticojejunostomy, although in practice this is rarely done.[14, 15]

11. INTRAPERITONEAL BLADDER INJURY: correct answer e

Intraperitoneal bladder injuries usually follow a blunt direct blowout to the lower abdomen with a distended bladder. Intraperitoneal bladder injuries also occur frequently in penetrating injuries of the lower abdomen.

Extraperitoneal bladder injuries are associated with pelvic injuries in 95% of cases. Conversely, only 5% of all pelvic fractures present with bladder injury.

Patients with intraperitoneal bladder injuries might present with no symptoms initially, or just with hematuria or difficulty voiding, but if the diagnosis is delayed, patients experience fever, abdominal distention, ileus, and peritoneal signs.

The diagnosis is confirmed by retrograde urethrocystography or a computed tomographic cystogram. If a kidney or urethral injury is suspected, excretory urography should be performed before retrograde urethrocystographic examination of the bladder. The radiologic studies show extravasation of the contrast to the paracolic gutters, outlining loops of bowel, pooling of contrast under the liver or spleen, or a combination thereof.

Extraperitoneal bladder injuries present with extravasation of the contrast adjacent to the pubic symphysis but confined to the bladder base.

Intraperitoneal bladder injury treatment consists of primary repair of the bladder injury. One layer of full-thickness absorbable stitches is adequate. Multiple layers are necessary in patients with previous history of pelvic irradiation, chronic infection, or multiple previous bladder operations.

Extraperitoneal bladder injuries can be managed by simple urinary catheter drainage for 7 to 10 days. Cystography after this period should be repeated to verify resolution of the leakage.[14]

Quick Answers

1. C	5. B	9. B
2. A	6. A	10. E
3. B	7. D	11. E
4. A	8. B	

REFERENCES

1. Stoleting R: Pharmacology and Physiology in Anesthetic Practice, 3rd ed. Philadelphia: JB Lippincott, 1999, pp 692–702.
2. Nyhus L, Baker R, Fischer J: Mastery of Surgery, 3rd ed. Boston: Little, Brown, 1997, p 310.
3. Sabiston D: The Biological Basis of Modern Surgical Practice, 15th ed. Philadelphia: WB Saunders, 1997, p 309.
4. Sabiston D: The Biological Basis of Modern Surgical Practice, 15th ed. Philadelphia: WB Saunders, 1997.
5. Cameron JL: Current Surgical Therapy, 6th ed. St. Louis: CV Mosby, 1998.
6. Marino PL: The ICU Book, 2nd ed. Baltimore: Williams & Wilkins, 1998.
7. Dean RH, Yao JST, Brewster DC: Current Diagnosis and Treatment in Vascular Surgery. Norwalk, CT: Appleton & Lange, 1995.
8. Frick EJ: Outcome of blunt thoracic aortic injury in a level I trauma center: An 8-year review. J Trauma 43:844–851, 1997.

9. Capan LM, Miller SM: Initial evaluation and resuscitation. Anesthesiol Clin North Am 1996.
10. American College of Surgeons: Advanced Trauma Life Support, 6th ed. Chicago: American College of Surgeons, 1997, pp 177–178.
11. Sabiston D: The Biological Basis of Modern Surgical Practice, 15th ed. Philadelphia: WB Saunders, 1997, pp 1410–1411.
12. Skandalakis JE, Skandalakis PN, Skandalakis LJ: Surgical Anatomy and Technique, A Pocket Manual, 2nd ed. New York: Springer, 1999.
13. Schwartz SI: Principle of Surgery, 7th ed. New York: McGraw-Hill, 1999.
14. Feliciano DV, Moore EE, Mattox KL: Trauma, 3rd ed. Stamford, CT: Appleton & Lange, 1998.
15. Townsend CM, Sabiston DC, eds: Sabiston Textbook of Surgery: The Biological Basis of Modern Surgical Practice, 16th ed. Philadelphia: WB Saunders, 2001.

NOTES

Endocrine

QUESTIONS

1. The external branch of the superior laryngeal nerve contains the motor fibers for which of the following muscles?
   a. Sternohyoid muscle
   b. Cricothyroid muscle
   c. Sternothyroid muscle
   d. Mylohyoid muscle
   e. Thyrohyoid muscle
2. A 50-year-old white man experiences diarrhea, multiple peptic ulcers, and a prolonged QT interval. What is the most appropriate surgical treatment for this patient?
   a. Whipple procedure
   b. Distal pancreatectomy
   c. Adrenalectomy
   d. Subtotal parathyroidectomy with reimplantation
   e. Thyroidectomy
   f. Pituitary adenoma resection
3. When performing a parotidectomy for a pleomorphic adenoma, all of the following statements are true except:
   a. This tumor is more common in women.
   b. The auriculotemporal nerve is the nerve most commonly injured.
   c. Frey syndrome (gustatory sweating) is a common complication.
   d. Superficial parotidectomy is an effective treatment.

e. Microscopically, these tumors do not have a true capsule.

4. The embryologic origin of the inferior parathyroid gland is the:
   a. Ultimobranchial body
   b. First pharyngeal pouch
   c. Second pharyngeal pouch
   d. Third pharyngeal pouch
   e. Fourth pharyngeal pouch

5. A 4-year-old child presents to the clinic with a family history of multiple endocrine neoplasia type 2A. Further investigations confirm this diagnosis and that the child has the *ret* mutation. Considering this patient's disease, choose the correct answer:
   a. You expect to find mucosal neuromas and marfanoid appearance.
   b. The child is at high risk for pancreatic cancer.
   c. You should recommend a prophylactic thyroidectomy at age 5.
   d. The child is at high risk for parathyroid carcinoma.
   e. Molecular genetic analysis probably shows a k-*ras* mutation.

6. Which is the most common site of extra-adrenal pheochromocytoma?
   a. Duodenum
   b. Inferior pole of the kidney
   c. Para-aortic area
   d. Parasplenic area
   e. Peripancreatic area

7. A 29-year-old white woman complains of a palpable mass in the right side of the neck. Physical examination reveals a palpable, round, mobile, nontender mass measuring approximately 2 cm

medial to the sternocleidomastoid muscle and lateral to the thyroid cartilage. Fine-needle aspiration is performed and shows a lymph node architecture with the presence of thyroid tissue. Which is the most appropriate initial approach for this patient?

a. Observation and follow-up in 1 month
b. Excisional biopsy of the lymph node
c. Thyroid profile, ultrasonography, and nuclear scan
d. Right modified radical neck dissection
e. Total thyroidectomy

8. Regarding papillary and follicular carcinoma of the thyroid, which one of the following is the incorrect statement?
   a. Papillary carcinoma is the most common thyroid cancer and is common in young patients.
   b. Follicular carcinoma of the thyroid exhibits hematogenous spread and has a worse prognosis than do papillary carcinomas.
   c. Papillary carcinomas usually present with lymphatic spread, and prophylactic modified radical neck dissection is appropriate in the treatment of these tumors.
   d. Radioactive therapy with ^{131}I is indicated for residual disease after surgery, distant metastases, and recurrent thyroid cancer.
   e. The treatment of papillary and follicular carcinoma consists mainly of near-total or total thyroidectomy.

9. Parathyroid hormone raises serum calcium levels, doing all of the following except:
   a. Stimulating vitamin D production
   b. Increasing renal tubular reabsorption of calcium

c. Decreasing renal tubular absorption of phosphate
d. Increasing bone reabsorption of calcium
e. Parathyroid hormone has a direct effect on bone, kidneys, and gut, leading to increased serum calcium concentration.

10. Regarding parathyroid cancer, which one of the following statements is true?
    a. It is a frequent cause of hyperparathyroidism.
    b. Most patients present with hypercalcemia but normal parathyroid hormone levels.
    c. The histopathologic criteria to differentiate parathyroid adenoma and parathyroid carcinoma are well defined.
    d. Parathyroid cancer is associated with multiple endocrine neoplasia type 1.
    e. Localizing studies are mandatory before neck exploration.

11. What is the most appropriate treatment for parathyroid cancer?
    a. Resect all four glands.
    b. Resect three glands and a portion of the fourth.
    c. Resect en bloc the involved gland and ipsilateral thyroid lobe.
    d. Resect en bloc the involved gland, followed by neck irradiation.
    e. Resect en bloc the involved gland, followed by chemotherapy.

ANSWERS

1. THYROID ANATOMY: correct answer b

The external branch of the superior laryngeal nerve is vulnerable to injury during thyroidectomy. It contains the motor fibers to the cricothyroid muscle, which functions to maintain the tone of the true vocal cords; when this branch is paralyzed, the voice loses its timbre and focus. This may also cause voice fatigue and can be potentially disastrous for singers and orators. To prevent this injury, ligation of the superior thyroid artery should be performed close to the point of entrance into the thyroid gland.[1]

2. MULTIPLE ENDOCRINE NEOPLASIA TYPE 1: correct answer d

Multiple endocrine neoplasia type 1 was first described by Wermer in 1954. Patients usually have the "three Ps": *p*ancreatic tumors, *p*ituitary adenomas, and *p*arathyroid hyperplasia.

The treatment for sporadic gastrinoma consists of resection of the tumor. Even if localization of the tumor is negative, including ^{131}I pentetreotide scan, computed tomography of the abdomen, and pancreatic venous sampling, exploration of the abdomen is warranted. Conversely, few surgeons support mandatory exploratory laparotomy for gastrinomas associated with multiple endocrine neoplasia type 1.

Initial surgical treatment for these patients should be aimed at correction of the hypercalcemia. A subtotal 3.5 parathyroidectomy with reimplantation of the remaining half is recommended. Correction of the hypercalcemia improves control of the acid secretion. Abdominal exploration should be performed in these cases for single, isolated, resectable lesions.[2, 3]

3. PAROTID SURGERY: correct answer b

Approximately 75% to 85% of salivary gland neoplasms occur in the parotid gland, most of them benign. The most common of these is pleomorphic adenoma. The female-to-male ratio is 1.7:1. The parotid gland is a single anatomic entity through which the branches of the facial nerve pass. Approximately 80% of the parenchyma of the gland occupies the subcutaneous space lateral to the facial nerve, designated the *superficial lobe.* A thin layer of parotid tissue lies beneath the facial nerve adjacent to the masseter muscle and ascending ramus of the mandible (deep lobe). Most neoplasms arise superficial to the nerve. Microscopically, these tumors do not have a true capsule but compress around normal salivary gland tissue, frequently having microscopic excrescences into normal tissue. Recurrence is thought to arise from these small islands of tumor, which may be left behind at operation, especially after enucleation.

The posterior branch of the greater auricular nerve is the nerve most commonly injured; after the nerve is identified running obliquely near the angle of the mandible, it is followed through the parotid gland to its posterior branch. This branch, which innervates the auricle and surrounding skin, is exposed completely after the more anterior branches are sacrificed. Subsequently, the nerve can be translocated posteriorly to avoid injury to it during identification of the main stem of the facial nerve. After superficial parotidectomy, permanent facial nerve injury occurs in about 1% and transient injury in about 30% of patients; 90% of the transient injuries resolve within 12 months. The most common complication after parotid surgery is Frey syndrome, characterized by dermal flushing and sweating of the skin preliminary to or during saliva production, sometimes accompanied by paresthesia at the surgical field. The syndrome presents 6 to 12 months after parotid surgery. This complication can be distressing because there is no satisfactory treatment. Pathophysiologically, the phenomenon is explained by the aberrant reinnervation of severed postganglionic sympathetic fibers that supply the sweat glands of the skin of the auriculotemporal region by the post-ganglionic secretomotor parasympathetic nerve fibers that innervate the parotid gland.[4, 5]

4. ANATOMY/EMBRYOLOGY: correct answer d

The inferior parathyroid gland arises from the third pharyngeal pouch as a proliferation of the dorsal wing cells, which comes to be on the posterior surface of the thyroid gland during the fourth to fifth week of development.

5. MULTIPLE ENDOCRINE NEOPLASIA SYNDROMES: correct answer c

Multiple endocrine neoplasia type 2 encompasses three distinct phenotypes: multiple endocrine neoplasia type 2, multiple endocrine neoplasia type 2B, and familial medullary carcinoma of the thyroid. Each condition manifests with C-cell hyperplasia, which progresses to multicentric medullary carcinoma of the thyroid. Patients with multiple endocrine neoplasia type 2A and multiple endocrine neoplasia type 2B also experience pheochromocytoma. Parathyroid hyperplasia-adenoma occurs with multiple endocrine neoplasia type 2A but is rare with multiple endocrine neoplasia type 2B. Multiple endocrine neoplasia type 2A and multiple endocrine neoplasia type 2B appear to be caused by a germline mutation of the RET proto-oncogene.

The multiple endocrine neoplasia type 2B syndrome is the only one with phenotypic characteristics: marfanoid appearance, mucosal neuromas, bony lesions, puffy lips, and megacolon.

The multiple endocrine neoplasia type 1 syndrome is associated with a menin gene defect, parathyroid hyperplasia, pancreatic tumors, and pituitary tumors.

Malignant transformation of a parathyroid gland is a truly rare phenomenon, and in most reported series of patients with primary hyperparathyroidism, the incidence of carcinoma is less than 1%.[6, 7]

6. PHEOCHROMOCYTOMA: correct answer c

Pheochromocytoma is a chromaffin tumor that arises from the neural crest cells. The most common site of pheochromocytoma is the medulla of the adrenal gland. The most common extra-adrenal gland site is the organ of Zuckerkandl, which consists of the neural tissue around the aorta at the level of the inferior mesenteric artery and the bifurcation. Sporadic pheochromocytoma can also be called the *disease of tens:* 10% occur in children, 10% are multiple, 10% are malignant, and 10% are bilateral.

Pheochromocytoma is found in patients with multiple endocrine neoplasia types 2A and 2B. In contrast to sporadic pheochromocytoma, these tumors are usually bilateral and malignant. The diagnosis is made by measuring epinephrine and norepinephrine levels and their metabolites metanephrine and vanillylmandelic acid in the urine. The tumor can be localized with computed tomography of the abdomen, magnetic resonance imaging, or ^{131}I-metaiodobenzylguanidine (^{131}I-MIBG) scanning. ^{131}I-MIBG is selectively taken up by adrenergic tissues and is the most sensitive test to diagnose ectopic tumors.

The treatment consists of resection of the tumor, which can be done openly or laparoscopically. Preoperatively, patients should be prepared with α- and β-blockers. Intraoperatively, the tumor should be manipulated as little as possible to avoid catecholamine release. The 2-year survival rate for patients with malignant pheochromocytoma is 30% to 40%. Metastases are common to bone, lymph nodes, liver, and lung.[8, 9]

7. THYROID CANCER: correct answer c

The initial approach for such patients is a full thyroid work-up, which includes fine-needle aspiration, thyroid profile and calcitonin level, thyroid ultrasonography, and a thyroid scan. If any of these studies is positive for papillary or medullary carcinoma of the thyroid, total thyroidectomy with en bloc node resection and modified radical neck dissection should be performed. Both medullary and papillary carcinoma of the thyroid require modified radical neck dissection in the presence of clinical nodal disease.[8–10]

8. THYROID CARCINOMA: correct answer c

Papillary carcinoma is the most common type of thyroid cancer and carries the best prognosis. Dissemination occurs through the lymphatics. Surgery is the main therapy for papillary and follicular carcinomas. For small tumors (<1.5 cm), thyroid lobectomy can be performed for papillary carcinomas. For tumors larger than 1.5 cm, total thyroidectomy is the operation of choice. Follicular carcinomas are treated with a total or near-total thyroidectomy. Modified neck dissection should be performed only for positive clinical disease (palpable lymph nodes).

Radioactive therapy with ^{131}I should be carried out for inoperable disease, postoperative residual disease in the neck, distant metastases, recurrent thyroid cancer, and cervical node metastases.[3, 8, 9]

9. PARATHYROID: correct answer e

Parathyroid hormone is essential in calcium homeostasis. Calcium is increased by

Stimulating vitamin D production, indirectly increasing absorption of calcium in the GI tract
Increasing renal tubular absorption of calcium
Decreasing renal tubular absorption of phosphate (phosphaturic effect)
Promoting resorption of bone matrix by osteoclasts

Hypoparathyroidism, which is most commonly caused by accidental removal or injury of the parathyroid glands after neck dissection or thyroidectomy, presents with the following findings:

Decreased parathyroid hormone levels
Decreased serum calcium levels
Increased serum phosphate levels

Patients with hypoparathyroidism present with muscular fatigue and weakness as well as numbness, the Chvostek sign (a tap over the facial nerve in front of the ear elicits a contraction of the facial muscles and upper lip), and a Trousseau sign (inflation of a blood pressure cuff on the arm to a pressure higher than the patient's systolic pressure for 3 minutes elicits carpal spasm).

Conversely, primary hyperparathyroidism, the most common cause of which is a single parathyroid adenoma (80%), presents with the following findings:

Increased parathyroid hormone levels
Increased serum calcium levels
Decreased serum phosphate levels
Elevation of chloride-to-phosphate ratio (>33)
Hypercalciuria

Patients with hyperparathyroidism can present with urinary calculi due to hypercalciuria, osteitis fibrosa cystica, bone cysts and brown tumors, hypertension (10% to 25%), peptic ulcer disease, pancreatitis (1%), constipation, depression, fatigue, and muscle weakness.[8, 11]

10. PARATHYROID CARCINOMA: correct answer b

Parathyroid cancer is an infrequent cause of hyperparathyroidism, accounting for less than 1% of cases. Approximately 85% of patients with parathyroid cancer present with abnormal calcium and parathyroid hormone levels. The histologic criteria for malignancy are poorly defined. History, physical examination, and evidence of local or distant invasion may play a key role in differentiating between malignant and benign disease.

Multiple endocrine neoplasia types 1 and 2 are associated with hyperparathyroidism due to parathyroid hyperplasia or parathyroid adenoma.

Localizing studies, including computed tomography of the neck, magnetic resonance imaging, venous sampling, and nuclear medicine imaging, are not mandatory before neck exploration. The sensitivity of radiologic studies still ranges from 70% to 85% and should be ordered only when the diagnosis of parathyroid disease is in doubt.[8, 11]

11. PARATHYROID CARCINOMA: correct answer c

Surgery is the only curative treatment for parathyroid cancer. Irradiation and chemotherapy are not beneficial. The 5- and 10-year survival rates are 40% and 20%, respectively. The cause of death usually is not metastatic disease but complications associated with severe hypercalcemia.[8, 11, 12]

Quick Answers

1. B	5. C	9. E
2. D	6. C	10. B
3. B	7. C	11. C
4. D	8. C	

REFERENCES

1. Sabiston D: The Biological Basis of Modern Surgical Practice, 15th ed. Philadelphia: WB Saunders, 1997, p 620.
2. Ellison AC: Forty-year appraisal of gastrinoma. Ann Surg 222:511–524, 1995.
3. Cameron JL: Current Surgical Therapy, 6th ed. St. Louis: CV Mosby, 1998.
4. Leverstein H, van der Wal JE, Tiwari RM, et al: Surgical management of 246 previously untreated pleomorphic adenomas of the parotid gland. Br J Surg 84:399–403, 1997.
5. McGurk M: Parotid pleomorphic adenoma. Br J Surg 84:1491–1492, 1997.
6. Clark O: Textbook of Endocrine Surgery, 1st ed. Philadelphia: WB Saunders, 1997, pp 108–111.
7. Spearling M: Pediatric Endocrinology, 1st ed. Philadelphia: WB Saunders, 1996, pp 315–325.
8. Townsend CM, Sabiston DC, eds: Sabiston Textbook of Surgery: The Biological Basis of Modern Surgical Practice, 16th ed. Philadelphia: WB Saunders, 2001.
9. Schwartz SI: Principles of Surgery, 7th ed. New York: McGraw-Hill, 1999.
10. Feig BW, Berger DH, Fuhrman GM: The M.D. Anderson Surgical Oncology Handbook, 2nd ed. Philadelphia: Lippincott Williams & Wilkins, 1999.

11. Wilson JD, Foster DW, Kronenberg HM, Larsen PR: Williams Textbook of Endocrinology, 9th ed. Philadelphia: WB Saunders, 1998.
12. Abeloff MD: Clinical Oncology, 2nd ed. New York: Churchill Livingstone, 2000.

NOTES

Peripheral Vascular and Cardiothoracic Surgery

QUESTIONS

1. A 24-year-old nonsmoking medical student presents with a 5-hour history of right pleuritic chest pain and dyspnea. The chest pain is described as moderate at onset and later as a "steady ache." The episode occurred while the patient was at rest. Physical findings include decreased movements of the chest wall, a hyperresonant percussion note, and decreased breath sounds of the right hemithorax. A chest radiograph confirms your suspicion of a spontaneous pneumothorax of the hemithorax of approximately 20%. Computed tomography of the chest reveals a single apical bulla 1 cm in diameter. A chest tube is placed without any complications, and symptoms improve. This is the second episode on the same side in the last 3 years. Definitive management of this patient includes which of the following interventions?
   a. Instillation of sclerosing agents through the chest tube in the absence of air leak
   b. Thoracoscopy through a single chest port with resection of the bulla and pleurodesis by mechanical pleural abrasion or insufflation of talc
   c. Video-assisted thoracoscopic surgery with multiple chest ports with resection of the bulla and pleurodesis

d. A limited axillary approach that spares the thoracic muscles (limited thoracotomy) with resection of the bulla and pleurodesis
e. Discharge of the patient home after removal of chest tube and radiographic evidence of no pneumothorax

2. Regarding splenic artery aneurysms, which of the following statements is correct?
   a. Splenic aneurysms are the second most common intra-abdominal aneurysm.
   b. They should always be resected.
   c. Part of the treatment includes splenectomy.
   d. Pregnant women have a low risk of rupture because of the intra-abdominal compression effect of the fetus.
   e. Most splenic aneurysms are diagnosed because of associated symptoms.

3. Which of the following asymptomatic patients requires surgical intervention?
   a. A 65-year-old with 2-cm popliteal artery aneurysm
   b. A 60-year-old with 4-cm thoracic aneurysm
   c. A 40-year-old with 2-cm subclavian aneurysm
   d. A 70-year-old with 4-cm abdominal aortic aneurysm
   e. An 80-year-old with 2.5-cm splenic artery aneurysm

4. A 67-year-old man underwent femoropopliteal bypass surgery with a saphenous vein graft because of resting pain in his right lower extremity 10 years before. He comes back to see you because of recurrence of the pain for the last week. Which is the most common cause of long-term failure of a peripheral vascular bypass graft?
   a. Technical error
   b. Atherosclerosis of the graft

c. Intimal hyperplasia
d. Aneurysm formation
e. Fibrosis of the graft

5. When comparing the retroperitoneal approach to the transabdominal approach for the repair of an elective aortic aneurysm, which of the following statements is false?
   a. Patients of American Society of Anesthesiologists (ASA) class IV who undergo aortic reconstruction with the retroperitoneal approach have a significant reduction in postoperative pain and in GI and cardiac complications.
   b. Operative time and blood loss are greater with the transabdominal approach.
   c. There are no differences in the incidence of pulmonary complications with either approach.
   d. There are no differences in the incidence of incisional hernias with either approach.
   e. There is no difference in perioperative mortality between the retroperitoneal and transabdominal approaches.

6. All of the following are known effects of cigarette smoking on atherogenesis except:
   a. Increased heart rate and blood pressure
   b. Increased endothelium-derived nitric oxide production
   c. Increased circulation of free fatty acids
   d. Increased permeability of the vessel walls to lipids
   e. Decreased cell synthesis of prostacyclin and increased production of thromboxane

7. Which of the following is the most common symptom at presentation reported by patients with lung cancer?
   a. Asymptomatic

b. Cough
c. Hemoptysis
d. Weight loss
e. Dyspnea

8. A 55-year-old white man presents to your clinic with the diagnosis of lung cancer. He complains of nausea, constipation, polydipsia, lethargy, and occasionally confusion. Physical examination reveals decreased deep tendon reflexes and cardiac arrhythmia. His laboratory test results show hypercalcemia. Which of the following tumors is most commonly associated with this patient's paraneoplastic endocrine syndrome?
   a. Small cell carcinoma
   b. Squamous cell carcinoma
   c. Adenocarcinoma
   d. Large cell carcinoma
   e. Bronchioalveolar carcinoma

9. Which one of the following is the most common paraneoplastic endocrine syndrome associated with lung cancer?
   a. Hypercalcemia (PTH-like syndrome)
   b. Cushing syndrome
   c. Syndrome of inappropriate antidiuretic hormone production
   d. Elevated β-human chorionic gonadotropin levels
   e. Eaton-Lambert syndrome

10. A 28-year-old white woman is referred from a community hospital for recurrent lung infections since childhood. Further investigation (computed tomography) reveals a pulmonary sequestration. From where does the blood supply to the sequestered parenchyma most frequently come?
   a. Pulmonary artery

b. Bronchial arteries
c. Aorta
d. Subclavian artery
e. Intercostal artery

11. Which is the most common mediastinal primary tumor in adults?
    a. Lymphoma
    b. Neuroblastoma
    c. Thymoma
    d. Teratoma
    e. Intrathoracic goiter

12. Which of the following characteristics of Buerger disease (thromboangiitis obliterans) is true?
    a. It is most commonly observed in young non-smoking females.
    b. It affects mainly the large arteries of the upper extremities.
    c. The histopathologic feature of the disease is the involvement of all layers of the vessel wall.
    d. Vascular reconstructive surgery is the main therapy.
    e. It tends to occur diffusely, with no skip lesions in the segment involved.

13. A 2-year-old boy comes to the clinic with the diagnosis of pulmonary hypertension. Which of the following is not associated with this disease?
    a. Patent ductus arteriosus
    b. Tetralogy of Fallot
    c. Ventricular septal defect
    d. Atrial septal defect
    e. Eisenmenger disease

14. Which one of the following is the best conduit for coronary artery bypass graft?
    a. Radial artery
    b. Right gastroepiploic artery

c. Saphenous vein
d. Internal mammary artery
e. Inferior epigastric artery

15. Regarding cardiac surgery, which one of the following is the correct statement?
   a. Coronary double vessel disease is an absolute indication for coronary bypass surgery.
   b. Left main coronary artery disease can be treated with stents.
   c. The mortality rate for coronary bypass surgery is approximately 10%.
   d. Mitral valve repair has a high failure rate, and mitral valve replacement should be performed whenever possible.
   e. Surgical intervention for aortic valve stenosis is warranted when the peak systolic gradient across the valve is more than 50 mmHg or the cross-sectional area of the valve is smaller than 1 cm^2.

16. An 80-year-old man comes into the emergency room with lower abdominal pain, bloody stools, and fever. Past medical history is significant for extensive vascular disease, including coronary artery disease, status/post (s/p) coronary artery bypass 10 years earlier, and s/p abdominal aortic aneurysms repair 20 years ago. On physical examination, he is slightly tachycardic (110 beats per minute) and hypotensive (blood pressure, 89/50). His abdomen is slightly tender in the lower quadrants, and his stools are Hemoccult-positive. Computed tomography of the abdomen reveals an aortoenteric fistula. Which one of the following statements is correct regarding this condition?
   a. The mortality rate is nearly 100%.
   b. Most of the fistulas occur between the aorta and the ileum.

c. Fistulas usually involve the proximal suture line of the aortic graft.
d. The treatment of choice is takedown of the fistula and graft replacement in the same position.
e. Primary aortoenteric fistulas are more common than secondary aortoenteric fistulas.

17. Regarding compartment syndrome, which one of the following statements is correct?
    a. The leg is divided into two compartments: anterior and posterior.
    b. The most common affected compartment is the posterior.
    c. The earliest manifestation of acute compartment syndrome is elevated tissue pressure.
    d. The peak time of symptoms appears to be 6 to 8 hours after the insult.
    e. Patients with compartment pressures greater than 15 mmHg should undergo fasciotomy.

ANSWERS

1. SPONTANEOUS PNEUMOTHORAX: correct answer b

Primary spontaneous pneumothorax typically occurs in tall, thin men between the ages of 10 and 30 years and rarely occurs in persons older than age 40. Smoking cigarettes increases the risk by a factor of 20 in a dose-dependent manner. A subpleural bulla is found in nearly all patients. The average rate of recurrence is 30%, and most recurrences are within 6 months to 2 years after the initial pneumothorax. Supplemental oxygen accelerates by a factor of 4 the reabsorption of air by the pleura, which occurs at a rate of 2% per day in patients breathing room air.

Interventions are recommended to prevent recurrences after the second ipsilateral pneumothorax. Patients who plan to continue activities that increase the risk of complications from a pneumothorax (e.g., flying or diving) should undergo preventive treatment after the first episode. These measures include instillation of sclerosing agents through chest tubes in the absence of air leaks, although this is associated with a recurrence rate of 8% to 25%, which is higher than the rate associated with other available methods. Thoracoscopy through a single chest port performed under direct visualization allows the resection of small apical bullae (<2 cm in diameter) and pleurodesis by mechanical pleural abrasion or insufflation of talc. The treatment of patients found at thoracoscopy to have bullae >2 cm in diameter can be switched to video-assisted thoracoscopic surgery or thoracotomy. The success rate for thoracoscopy with insufflation of talc is approximately 97%, with a recurrence rate of 5% to 9%. Video-assisted thoracoscopic surgery with multiple chest ports allows wide visualization of the pleural space for the resection of bullae and pleurodesis. Recurrence rates vary from 2% to 14% as compared with a range of 0% to 7% for limited thoracotomy. An approach that uses thoracoscopy through a single chest port is recommended; patients found to have large apical bullae should be switched to video-assisted thoracoscopic surgery or a limited thoracotomy.[1]

2. SPLENIC ARTERY ANEURYSMS: correct answer a

Although infrequent, splenic artery aneurysms are the second most common intra-abdominal aneurysm, the aorta being the most common site of occurrence. Patients are usually asymptomatic, and the diagnosis is usually an incidental finding.

Some patients complain of left upper quadrant abdominal pain, fullness, nausea, and vomiting.

Neither old patients without symptoms nor small aneurysms (<2 cm) are indications for surgical intervention. Conversely, women of childbearing age should undergo resection of splenic aneurysms because of the high mortality rate associated with rupture.

Splenectomy can be avoided when these aneurysms are distal to the hilum. Splenectomy is indicated when aneurysms are proximal to the hilum or when rupture occurs.[2, 3]

3. ANEURYSMS: correct answer a

Popliteal artery aneurysms always require surgical intervention: 50% of patients have bilateral aneurysms, and 75% have aneurysms in another site of the body.

Clinically, most patients with popliteal artery aneurysm present with pain and a cold lower extremity due to thrombosis of the aneurysm.

Because of the risk of limb loss, surgical correction is indicated solely by the presence of a popliteal artery aneurysm.

For thoracic and aortic aneurysms, the cutoff for repair is 5 cm or when they increase more than 0.5 cm in 6 months. Splenic aneurysms should be resected in young patients, mainly in women of childbearing age because of the high mortality rate in the mother and fetus (approximately 70%) that is associated with rupture.

Subclavian aneurysms should be resected when symptomatic and when bigger than 2.5 times the normal diameter of the vessel.[3, 4]

4. VASCULAR SURGERY: correct answer c

Intimal hyperplasia is the most common cause of long-term graft failure, followed by atherosclerosis, fibrosis of the graft due to side branches ligation, and aneurysm formation.

Technical error is the most common cause of early graft dysfunction.

Primary patency of the femoropopliteal saphenous vein grafts is approximately 80% to 90%. Long-term patency ranges from 40% to 50%. Intimal hyperplasia was initially described by Carren, who noticed thickening of the venous grafts after placing them under arterial pressure. Fibrointimal hyperplasia follows the conversion of normally quiescent myointimal and medial smooth muscle cells into active fibroblasts.[3, 5, 6]

5. ABDOMINAL AORTIC ANEURYSM REPAIR: correct answer b

Patients of ASA class IV who undergo aortic reconstruction with the retroperitoneal approach experience a significant reduction in postoperative pain and in GI and cardiac complications, which results in a shortened hospital stay and cost savings. Although operative time and blood loss are greater with the retroperitoneal approach, there is no difference in the incidence of pulmonary complications or incisional hernias. There is no difference between the retroperitoneal and transabdominal groups in the perioperative mortality or survival rates at 40 months. In patients of ASA class IV, abdominal aortic operations can be more safely and economically performed with the retroperitoneal approach.

The retroperitoneal approach avoids the midline incision and the associated bowel dilation and rectus spasm that may cause severe discomfort that can hinder patient mobilization, pulmonary toilet, and resumption of GI tract function.

The technical advantages of the retroperitoneal approach include the avoidance of adhesions from prior abdominal operations, the easier exposure in patients who are obese, the improved exposure of the aortic "neck" in large aneurysms, the easier juxtarenal and suprarenal aortic control, the safer repair of inflammatory aneurysms, and the greater safety in patients with certain renal vascular anomalies. The cited physiologic advantages of the retroperitoneal approach include decreased postoperative ileus, decreased third-space fluid loss, reduced hypothermia, fewer hemodynamic stresses, decreased pulmonary compromise, faster recovery, and fewer overall complications. These potential physiologic benefits are thought to result from the fact that the peritoneal cavity is not violated and that its contents are not manipulated, which thereby results in diminished heat and evaporative losses, less third-space fluid loss, decreased postoperative pain, and reduced compromise of pulmonary and GI function. The potential disadvantages of the retroperitoneal approach include poor access to the right renal artery and inability to visualize the left colon after revascularization.[7]

6. ATHEROSCLEROSIS: correct answer b

Vascular injury and thrombus formation are the major events in the formation and progression of the atherosclerotic lesion. Carbon monoxide causes increased permeability of the vessel wall to lipids. Nicotine produces increased levels of circulating free fatty acids, which increase the intracellular lipid deposition. It also decreases cell synthesis of prostacyclin, the most potent inhibitor of platelet aggregation, and promotes the production of thromboxane, which stimulates platelet aggregation.

Endothelium-derived nitric oxide and prostacyclin inhibit several processes that promote the development of an atherosclerotic plaque. Nitric oxide is a vasodilator that inhibits platelet aggregation and the proliferation of vascular smooth muscle cells and suppresses the generation of oxygen free radicals, decreasing endothelial injury.[8, 9]

7. LUNG CANCER: correct answer b

Cough	45%–75%
Weight loss	20%–70%
Dyspnea	40%–60%
Chest pain	30%–45%
Hemoptysis	25%–35%

8. LUNG CANCER/PARANEOPLASTIC SYNDROME: correct answer b

Hypercalcemia occurs in 10% to 12.5% of all patients with lung cancer. Approximately 10% to 15% of these cases are caused by a secretion of a parathyroid hormone–related protein. In contrast to all the other paraneoplastic syndromes (which are more common with small cell lung cancer), this one is more common with squamous cell lung cancer.[10, 11]

9. PARANEOPLASTIC SYNDROMES/LUNG CANCER: correct answer c

Syndrome of inappropriate antidiuretic hormone production: 27%
Hypercalcemia (parathyroid hormone–like syndrome): 12.5%
Cushing syndrome: 6%
Elevated β-human chorionic gonadotropin levels: 2%
Hypoglycemia: $<1\%$[10]

10. PULMONARY SEQUESTRATION: correct answer c

During development, a portion of the lung may be isolated from the remainder of the lung and receive its blood supply from an aberrant branch of the aorta instead of from the pulmonary artery.

There are (1) intralobar sequestrations that rest within a lobe and do not have their own visceral pleural envelope but usually communicate with the tracheobronchial tree, producing a cystic appearance and (2) extralobar sequestrations, a less common entity in which the sequestered lung is enclosed by a separate pleural envelope.[10]

11. MEDIASTINAL TUMOR: correct answer c

Among 400 patients with mediastinal tumors reported by Davis and associates, thymic neoplasms were the most common primary tumor, occurring in 17% of cases; lymphoma occurred in 16% of cases, neurogenic tumors in 14%, and germ cell tumors in 11%. The thyroid gland is not considered a mediastinal organ.[10]

12. THROMBOANGIITIS OBLITERANS: correct answer c

Buerger disease is an inflammatory vasculopathy occurring in medium-sized and small arteries of young male smokers. The disease is extremely rare in females and is not observed in nonsmokers. The lesions occur in the upper and lower extremities, in veins as well as arteries, tending to appear in a localized segmental fashion, with normal vessel segments interposed between involved segments. The histopathologic features are those of a panarteritis, involving all layers of the vessel wall. Vascular reconstructive surgery is not feasible because the involvement of small vessels makes it difficult to locate suitable outflow sites for bypass grafts.

Therapy is directed against the inciting effects of tobacco, with complete arrest of the process once smoking has been abandoned.[10]

13. CONGENITAL CARDIAC DEFECTS: correct answer b

Tetralogy of Fallot is a right-to-left shunt and is not associated with pulmonary hypertension, as opposed to the other choices (left-to-right shunts leading to Eisenmenger syndrome).[12]

14. CARDIOVASCULAR: correct answer d

The internal mammary artery has been shown to be the best conduit for coronary artery bypass surgery. This vessel appears to be virtually immune to atherosclerosis and has 90% potency in 5 years. Patients in whom the internal mammary artery is used as a conduit have a decreased risk of myocardial infarction, late death, and reoperation, and the clinical benefit persists for up to 20 years.

The saphenous vein is a good conduit, especially in emergency cases in which one surgeon works in the chest and another quickly harvests the saphenous vein in the leg. Many studies have shown that early occlusion of the saphenous vein conduit occurs in 8% to 12% of cases. Furthermore, the accelerated atherosclerosis can compromise this conduit in less than 5 years.

The radial artery can also be used as a conduit for coronary artery bypass. Special attention must be paid to avoid acute vasospasm. Minimal manipulation, calcium channel blockers, and papaverine are all helpful in increasing the early patency of this conduit. Indeed, a patency of 84% has been reported when this conduit is used.

In special cases, the right gastroepiploic artery or the inferior epigastric artery can be used as a conduit for coronary artery bypass. Further studies are necessary to evaluate the long-term patency of these vessels.[6, 13]

15. CARDIAC SURGERY: correct answer e

Surgical intervention for aortic stenosis is indicated when patients present with symptoms (e.g., dyspnea, syncope), a peak systolic gradient across the valve of more than 50 mmHg, or a cross-sectional area of 0.8 to 1.0 cm^2, which indicates moderate to severe aortic stenosis.

Indications for coronary artery bypass include triple-vessel disease, left main disease, and refractory cases or complications after percutaneous coronary angioplasty.

Mitral valve repair is a successful procedure (90% of patients are free of symptoms for 5 years) and should be attempted whenever possible. Patients who undergo mitral valve repair do not require chronic anticoagulation.[6, 13]

16. AORTOENTERIC FISTULAS: correct answer c

Secondary aortoenteric fistulas are an unusual late postoperative complication (0.9%) with repair of abdominal aortic aneurysms, associated with a mortality rate exceeding 50%. Most fistulas occur at the level of the proximal suture line and almost always involve the duodenum. The treatment of choice is resection of the graft followed by an extra-anatomic bypass.[3, 6]

17. VASCULAR–ACUTE COMPARTMENT SYNDROME: correct answer c

The earliest manifestation of acute compartment syndrome is elevated tissue pressure. Signs and symptoms occur after tissue pressure has been elevated beyond a critical period. The first clinical symptom is pain, followed by decreased passive range of motion due to pain, paresthesias, and absence of pulse. When a distal pulse is obliterated, tissue has most likely been damaged irreversibly. The onset of symptoms can occur from 2 hours to days after the initial insult. The peak time of appearance of symptoms is between 15 and 30 hours.

The literature is not unanimous in the normal compartment pressure values, ranging from 0 to 16 mmHg. Pressures greater than 25 mmHg are considered abnormal but do not necessarily precipitate a compartment syndrome. The decision to perform fasciotomy should be based on clinical signs and symptoms.

Extremities are quick to develop compartment syndrome because of their confined environment, especially lower extremities. The leg is divided into three compartments: anterior, which is the most susceptible to compartment syndrome; posterior, which is subdivided into superficial and deep compartments; and lateral.[5, 14]

Quick Answers

1. B	7. B	13. B
2. A	8. B	14. D
3. A	9. C	15. E
4. C	10. C	16. C
5. B	11. C	17. C
6. B	12. C	

REFERENCES

1. Sahn S, Heffner J: Spontaneous pneumothorax. N Engl J Med 342:868–874, 2000.
2. Way LW: Current Surgical Diagnosis and Treatment, 4th ed. Norwalk, CT: Appleton & Lange, 1998.

3. Dean RH, Yao JST, Brewster DC: Current Diagnosis and Treatment in Vascular Surgery. Norwalk, CT: Appleton & Lange, 1995.
4. Locati P: Popliteal aneurysms: current management and outcome. Minerva Cardioangiol 47:145–155, 1999.
5. Cameron JL: Current Surgical Therapy, 6th ed. St. Louis: CV Mosby, 1998.
6. Townsend CM, Sabiston DC, eds: Sabiston Textbook of Surgery: The Biological Basis of Modern Surgical Practice, 16th ed. Philadelphia: WB Saunders, 2001.
7. Kirby LB, Rosenthal D, Atkins CP, et al: Comparison between the transabdominal and retroperitoneal approaches for aortic reconstruction in patients at high risk. J Vasc Surg 30:400–406, 1999.
8. Schwartz SI: Principles of Surgery, 7th ed. New York: McGraw-Hill, 1999, pp 931–933.
9. Rutherford RB: Vascular Surgery, 5th ed. Philadelphia: WB Saunders, 2000, pp 333–338.
10. Shields TW, LoCicero J, Ponn RB, eds: General Thoracic Surgery, 5th ed. Philadelphia: Lippincott Williams & Wilkins, 2000, pp 1269–1275.
11. Pass HI: Lung Cancer: Principles and Practice, 2nd ed. Philadelphia: Lippincott Williams & Wilkins, 2000, pp 525–527.
12. Sabiston D: Textbook of Surgery, 15th ed. Philadelphia: WB Saunders, 1997.
13. Braunwald E: Heart Disease: A Textbook of Cardiovascular Medicine, 6th ed. Philadelphia: WB Saunders, 2001.
14. Roberts JR: Clinical Procedures in Emergency Medicine, 3rd ed. Philadelphia: WB Saunders, 1998.

NOTES

Pediatric Surgery

QUESTIONS

1. A 2-year-old child is brought by his mother to the pediatric clinic because of an abdominal mass and fever. Other clinical findings include macroglossia, linear ear creases, and hemi-hypertrophy. Computed tomography shows a retroperitoneal mass arising from the left kidney. Besides this tumor, what other kind of tumor is this patient predisposed to?
   a. Hepatoblastoma
   b. Neuroblastoma
   c. Retinoblastoma
   d. Osteosarcoma
   e. Rhabdomyosarcoma
2. A 10-year-old healthy boy comes into your office complaining of a lump on his right thigh, which was noticed 6 weeks ago. He says that 2 months ago he had a "pulled muscle" on that leg and since then he has had this mass, which is growing. On physical examination, there is a well-circumscribed mass on the anterior aspect of his right thigh, measuring about 6 cm in its greater diameter, hard, and barely mobile. The first step toward diagnosis is:
   a. Fine-needle aspiration
   b. Tru-Cut biopsy
   c. Magnetic resonance imaging
   d. Incisional biopsy
   e. Excisional biopsy

3. Which of the following is the correct statement?
   a. Omphalocele is an anterior abdominal wall defect lateral to the umbilicus.
   b. Gastroschisis is more often associated with other congenital anomalies than omphalocele.
   c. The prognosis of omphalocele is related to the size of the defect.
   d. Prenatal diagnosis of abdominal wall defects is difficult, but when the diagnosis is established, cesarean section is mandatory.
   e. In most babies with gastroschisis, the abdomen fails to close primarily.

4. Regarding necrotizing enterocolitis, which one of the following is the correct statement?
   a. Pneumatosis intestinalis is an indication for exploratory laparotomy.
   b. Patients with extensive involvement from the duodenum to the midtransverse colon require immediate aggressive bowel resection.
   c. Mortality is not associated with prematurity and birthweight.
   d. Liver hemorrhage is usually a lethal complication.
   e. Bowel stricture is a common complication after necrotizing enterocolitis and occurs most frequently at the jejunum.

5. Regarding malrotation and midgut volvulus, which is the correct statement?
   a. They are rarely associated with other congenital anomalies.
   b. The cecum is usually found in the left lower quadrant.
   c. Plain films of the abdomen show an airless colon, and an upper GI imaging series demonstrates an obstruction at the level of the proximal jejunum.

d. Volvulus undergoes detorsion in a clockwise direction.
e. Midgut volvulus can occur at any time throughout one's life.

6. Which one of the following is correct regarding the care of the pediatric surgical patient?
   a. Newborns shiver more easily than adults because they store relatively little subcutaneous fat.
   b. Newborns should have a urinary output of approximately 0.5 mL/kg/hr.
   c. The maintenance fluid of choice in a newborn is 10% dextrose in 0.25% normal saline.
   d. In neonates, the cellular immune response is impaired, but the humoral immune response is fully mature.
   e. The arterial partial pressure of oxygen (Pao_2) in a newborn from blood obtained from a radial artery is approximately 90 to 100 mmHg.

7. Regarding the nutritional requirements of the newborn, which one of the following statements is correct ?
   a. Parenteral alimentation should be implemented in all premature newborns due to their increased risk of necrotizing enterocolitis.
   b. Neonates require approximately 50 to 70 kcal/kg/day for growth.
   c. Low osmolar lactose-free formulas should be used in postoperative patients.
   d. Newborns require 4 to 5 g/kg/day of protein for growth.
   e. The ratio of nonprotein calorie per gram of nitrogen is maintained at 100:1 or less to avoid overfeeding.

8. Regarding intestinal atresia of the newborn, which of the following statements is true?
   a. Duodenal atresia usually occurs at the second portion of the duodenum, just distal to the ampulla of Vater.
   b. Approximately 60% to 70% of duodenal atresias are associated with Down syndrome.
   c. Treatment of duodenal atresia consists of end-to-end duodenoduodenostomy.
   d. Atresia of the jejunum is more common than atresia of the ileum and usually results from intrauterine vascular accidents to the mesenteric circulation.
   e. Bilious emesis, associated with a flat abdomen, usually occurs in newborns with intestinal atresia.

9. Which one of the following is the most common type of tracheoesophageal (TE) fistula?
   a. Esophageal atresia alone
   b. Esophageal atresia with proximal TE fistula
   c. H-type TE fistula without esophageal atresia
   d. Esophageal atresia with double TE fistula
   e. Esophageal atresia with distal TE fistula

ANSWERS

1. BECKWITH-WIEDEMANN SYNDROME: correct answer a

This syndrome is characterized by excessive intrauterine and postnatal growth, organomegaly, macroglossia, linear ear creases, omphalocele, umbilical defects, and hemihypertrophia. The risk of Wilms tumor is as high as 40% and is associated with a high risk of hepatoblastoma. Retinoblastoma is the most common malignant tumor affecting children, occurring as a sporadic mutation (RB1G) (60% of cases) or as an inherited condition. The genetic defect is the loss of heterozygosity at the RB gene locus that predisposes the child to retinoblastoma. The RB1 gene is located in the 13q14.1 region. The RB1 gene is a tumor suppressor gene that is also associated with osteosarcomas. Rhabdomyosarcoma is the most common malignant tumor of soft tissue in children.[1]

2. SOFT TISSUE SARCOMAS: correct answer b

Soft tissue sarcomas are uncommon malignancies. Genetic diseases such as neurofibromatosis, familial adenomatous polyposis, and Li-Fraumeni syndrome are associated with soft tissue sarcomas. Other predisposing factors may play a role in the development of the disease such as lymphedema, radiation, and chemicals (arsenic, polyvinyl chloride, 2,3,7,8-tetrachlorodibenzodioxin).

The degree of malignancy is graded (low, intermediate, or high) and is used as a prognostic factor along with the histologic type.

Tissue diagnosis is made with an excisional biopsy in tumors measuring less than 5 cm and with a Tru-Cut biopsy in tumors bigger than 5 cm. Incisional biopsy can also be considered for tumors measuring more than 5 cm. At present, magnetic resonance imaging is considered the imaging test of choice to diagnose soft tissue sarcomas. Fine-needle aspiration is not considered reliable for the diagnosis of soft tissue sarcomas.[2–4]

3. PEDIATRICS: correct answer c

Omphalocele is an umbilical ring defect associated with herniation of abdominal contents. The hernia sac is covered with peritoneum, and the prognosis is directly related to the size of the defect and to associated congenital anomalies, which are less common in babies with gastroschisis. Treatment is individualized for each patient. For small defects (smaller <2 cm), primary closure is the best treatment option. For larger defects, a polyester (Dacron) reinforced polymeric silicone (Silastic) silo is used to cover the viscera temporarily. The silo can be cut and reduced in size; the patient is then returned to the operating theater for formal closure of the abdominal wall.

Gastroschisis is a defect of the abdominal wall lateral to the umbilicus. No peritoneum covers the intestines, leading to the development of a thick exudative membrane over the bowel. Treatment consists of attempted primary closure of the defect, which is successful in 70% of cases.

Prenatal diagnosis of an abdominal wall defect is frequently performed with ultrasonography. Vaginal delivery is not contraindicated in the presence of abdominal wall defects.

4. PEDIATRICS: correct answer d

Liver hemorrhage is a serious complication in patients who undergo exploratory laparotomy for necrotizing enterocolitis. Massive fluid resuscitation, coagulopathy, and inadequate surgical technique are risk factors for this complication. The mortality rate associated with liver hemorrhage is approximately 85% and is due to the technical difficulties that surgeons face in controlling the bleeding.

Pneumatosis intestinalis itself is not an indication for laparotomy. Radiographic findings that suggest exploratory laparotomy are portal venous air and pneumoperitoneum. Clinical findings such as fever, an erythematous abdominal wall, persistent acidosis, and a decreased platelet count suggest that one proceed with exploration. Surgical treatment is individualized for each patient. Patients with extensive necrosis of the bowel from the duodenum to the midtransverse colon should be treated without any bowel resection initially. A "second look" operation 24 to 48 hours later should be performed for bowel viability. Most of these patients die from sepsis and sirds.

Mortality is associated with low birth weight and prematurity. Actually, almost 90% of cases of necrotizing enterocolitis are associated with these two conditions. The survival rate is approximately 80% without surgery, dropping to 60% after exploratory laparotomy.

Stenosis or stricture of the bowel occurs in approximately 10% to 25% of cases and is most frequent in the colon and ileum.[2]

5. PEDIATRICS: correct answer e

Anomalies of the intestinal rotation occur between the 5th and 12th weeks of gestational life. The small bowel is not fixed to the posterior wall, the colon is not fixed to the lateral abdominal walls, the cecum does not migrate from the upper abdomen to the right lower quadrant, and bands develop between the duodenum and the cecum. The bowel is sustained by a pedicle formed by the superior mesenteric artery and vein. Because of the abnormal bands, the bowel can rotate clockwise, leading to a midgut volvulus.

Diagnosis is made clinically. Patients usually present in the first week of life with bilious vomiting, abdominal distention, and abdominal tenderness. Plain films reveal a gasless colon, and an upper GI imaging series demonstrates an obstruction at the level of the second or third portion of the duodenum.

At the time of exploratory laparotomy, a counterclockwise rotation should be performed; abnormal bands among the cecum, duodenum, and jejunum should be resected; the colon should be placed on the left side of the abdomen; the cecum should be fixed near the sigmoid colon; and, finally, appendectomy should be performed. This operation is called the *Ladd procedure*.

Midgut volvulus occurs 85% of the time in the first week of life, but patients with malrotation can experience midgut volvulus at any point in their lives. This is why surgeons advocate exploratory laparotomy and Ladd's procedure at any time when malrotation is diagnosed.[2]

6. PHYSIOLOGY OF THE NEWBORN: correct answer c

The fluid of choice in newborns is D10 plus 0.25% normal saline for several reasons. D10 should be used because newborns tend to experience hypoglycemia and hypothermia because of their limited subcutaneous tissue and fat storage, lack of hair, and relatively large body surface area. Newborns have kidney tubular immaturity and a decreased glomerular filtration rate, which explains why 0.25% normal saline maintenance is used. A urinary output of 1 to 2 mL/kg/hr is considered appropriate for these patients.

Newborns do not shiver but respond to stress and cold by increasing their metabolic rate and oxygen consumption by mobilizing brown fat deposits from the axilla, neck, mediastinum, and perirenal area (nonshivering thermogenesis).

The humoral and cellular immune responses of neonates are immature. Impairment of leukocyte function and decreased levels of immunoglobulins make neonates more susceptible to infection.

Normal blood gas tension in newborns is different from that in adults because of shunting (foramen ovale, patent ductus). The Pao_2 above the ductus (sample obtained from the radial artery) is approximately 75 to 80 mmHg, and the Pao_2 below the ductus (sample obtained from the umbilical cord) should be approximately 60 mmHg.[2]

7. POSTOPERATIVE NUTRITION IN NEWBORNS: correct answer c

Low osmolar lactose-free formulas should be used after abdominal surgery because of the flattening of villi.

Neonates require approximately 120 kcal/kg/day, and the ratio of nonprotein calorie per gram of nitrogen should be kept at approximately 150:1.

A continuous drip of a solution containing 17% carbohydrates, 2 to 3.5 g/kg protein, and 4 g/kg fat emulsion administered as 10% or 20% should be able to deliver approximately 120 to 130 kcal/kg/day.

Enteral feedings should always be used when possible. Parenteral alimentation should be reserved for whenever the gut cannot be used, such as with necrotizing enterocolitis, severe gastroenteritis, thermal burns, and short gut syndrome. Prematurity itself is not a criterion for starting hyperalimentation unless the diagnosis of necrotizing enterocolitis has been established.[2]

8. DUODENAL ATRESIA: correct answer a

Duodenal atresia occurs at the second portion of the duodenum, usually distal to the ampulla of Vater. In 30% of cases of duodenal atresia, Down syndrome is present. Treatment consists of a side-to-side duodenoduodenostomy or duodenojejunostomy.

Ileal atresias are more common than jejunal atresias; both result from an intrauterine vascular accident to the mesenteric circulation.

Children with intestinal atresia usually present with bilious vomiting and abdominal distention. Babies with more proximal anomalies vomit earlier than those with distal obstruction. Intestinal atresias are rarely associated with other anomalies.[2]

9. TRACHEOESOPHAGEAL FISTULA: correct answer e

The most common type of esophageal atresia and TE fistula is called type C, wherein an esophageal atresia is associated with distal TE fistula. This occurs in 85% of cases, followed by proximal esophageal atresia without TE fistula (type A, 8% of cases), H-type TE fistula without esophageal atresia (type B, 4% of cases), and esophageal atresia associated with double TE fistula (type D, 2% of cases).[2]

Quick Answers

1. A	4. D	7. C
2. B	5. E	8. A
3. C	6. C	9. E

REFERENCES

1. Leenhard R: Clinical Oncology. Atlanta, GA, American Cancer Society, 2001, pp 577–585.
2. Townsend CM, Sabiston DC, eds: Sabiston Textbook of Surgery: The Biological Basis of

Modern Surgical Practice, 16th ed. Philadelphia: WB Saunders, 2001.

3. Schwartz SI: Principles of Surgery, 7th ed. New York: McGraw-Hill, 1999.
4. Cotran RS: Robbins Pathologic Basis of Disease, 6th ed. Philadelphia: WB Saunders, 1999.

NOTES

Transplantation

QUESTIONS

1. Regarding the immune system and transplantation, which of the following is the correct statement?
   a. Graft survival is the same in patients who undergo pancreatic transplantation with total human leukocyte antigen mismatch compared with patients who have one or more human leukocyte antigen matches.
   b. Liver recipients with a positive cross-match have worse outcomes than do patients with a negative cross-match.
   c. B cells play a major role in acute cellular rejection; T cells are the key cells in hyperacute rejection.
   d. Interleukin-2 is upregulated in acute rejection and in graft loss.
   e. Cytotoxic T-lymphocyte antigen 4 (CTLA-4) upregulates the immune system and is responsible for graft rejection.

2. What is the correct sequence of the vascular anastomosis when performing a liver transplantation?
   a. Suprahepatic vena cava, infrahepatic vena cava, portal vein, hepatic artery
   b. Portal vein, hepatic artery, suprahepatic vena cava, infrahepatic vena cava
   c. Hepatic artery, portal vein, infrahepatic vena cava, suprahepatic vena cava
   d. Hepatic artery, infrahepatic vena cava, suprahepatic vena cava, portal vein

   e. Infrahepatic vena cava, suprahepatic vena cava, hepatic artery, portal vein

3. What is the main factor limiting long-term survival in lung transplant recipients?
   a. Obliterative bronchiolitis
   b. Malignancy
   c. Respiratory failure
   d. Heart failure
   e. Cytomegalovirus

4. Acute allograft rejection involves mainly which of the following cells?
   a. B lymphocytes
   b. T lymphocytes
   c. Natural killer cells
   d. Macrophages
   e. Neutrophils

5. Regarding the major histocompatibility complex (MHC), which of the following statements is true?
   a. There are three different MHC class I molecules: human leukocyte antigen (HLA)-DP, HLA-DQ, HLA-DR.
   b. Class I MHC molecules are found in all cells of the body.
   c. Class II MHC molecules are found only in inactivated cells.
   d. HLA matching is essential in all solid organ transplantation.
   e. The function of MHC class I cells is the elimination of abnormal host cells.

6. Regarding immunosuppressive drugs, which of the following statements is true?
   a. Cyclosporine, an inhibitor of the production and release of interleukin-2 (IL-2), is exclusively metabolized and excreted by the kidneys.

b. FK506, another inhibitor of IL-2, is less nephrotoxic than cyclosporine.
c. Mycophenolate mofetil inhibits IL-1 production and release.
d. Rapamycin blocks IL-2 expression and production and works synergistically with cyclosporine and FK506.
e. OKT3 is a murine monoclonal antibody that reacts with the CD3 molecule on T lymphocytes.

7. Regarding the side effects of the immunosuppressive drugs, which one of the following statements is not true?
   a. Cyclosporine is nephrotoxic and hepatotoxic.
   b. FK506 can cause glucose intolerance and altered mental status.
   c. Diarrhea and thrombocytopenia are side effects of mycophenolate mofetil.
   d. Rapamycin is nephrotoxic and can cause hyperlipidemia.
   e. Fevers, nausea, vomiting, bronchospasm, and pulmonary edema can occur during OKT3 infusion.

8. Regarding viral infection and transplantation, which one of the following statements is incorrect?
   a. Herpes simplex virus hepatitis occurs late after solid organ transplantation, and most cases represent primary infection with the donor virus.
   b. Approximately 50% to 60% of transplant recipients shed Epstein-Barr virus asymptomatically.
   c. Half of the seropositive recipients of kidney transplantation from a donor who is

seropositive for cytomegalovirus (CMV) experience CMV infection if no prophylactic therapy is used.

d. Kaposi sarcoma is associated with human herpesvirus 8, and the mean time of onset after transplantation is 21 months.

e. Clinical manifestations of BK polyomavirus infection in patients after renal transplantation include hemorrhagic cystitis, ureteral strictures, and interstitial nephritis.

9. Regarding post-transplantation lymphoproliferative disorder (PTLD), which one of the following statements is incorrect?
   a. Epstein-Barr virus is implicated in the development of PTLD.
   b. PTLD is responsible for 20% of malignancies in kidney transplant patients.
   c. Extranodal involvement is present in 70% of cases and most times involves the GI tract, allograft, or central nervous system.
   d. The great majority of cases of PTLD are T-cell lymphomas.
   e. Initial treatment consists of reduction or withdrawal of immunosuppressive therapy and avoidance of antilymphocyte globulin therapy.

10. A 45-year-old man underwent cadaveric kidney transplantation. On postoperative day 2, his urinary output dropped and his creatinine serum levels rose from 1.3 mg/dL to 1.8 mg/dL. Regarding management, which one of the following statements is incorrect?
    a. The microscopic hallmark of acute cadaveric graft rejection is cellular infiltration.
    b. Immediate reoperation without delay for diagnostic studies is usually the only chance for salvaging a graft after arterial thrombosis.

c. The most common cause of acute cessation of urinary output in the immediate postoperative period is the presence of a blood clot in the bladder or urethral catheter.
d. Lymphoceles should always be drained.
e. Changes in urine volume may not occur initially with a necrosing ureter, which can contain urine flow for days before overt rupture.

ANSWERS

1. TRANSPLANT: correct answer d

IL-2 is secreted by T lymphocytes and upregulates the immune system through the proliferation and differentiation of T and B cells. Calcineurin inhibitors, such as cyclosporine, tacrolimus, and rapamycin, block or inhibit the production of IL-2, blunting the immune response. T cells play a major role in acute cellular graft rejection. Hyperacute rejection is caused by preformed antibodies, and T cells play a secondary role in this kind of immune response.

It has been shown that liver transplant recipients with a positive cross-match have the same outcome as patients with negative cross-match.

CTLA-4 (CD 152) is a cell surface protein that binds to CD80 and CD86 (ligands). This binding generates a negative regulatory signal and consequent downregulation of the immune system. Conversely, CD28, a molecule highly homologous to CTLA-4, binds to the same ligands (CD80 and CD86) and leads to upregulation of the immune response.[1–3]

2. LIVER TRANSPLANTATION: correct answer a

The implantation procedure begins with suprahepatic vena cava anastomosis followed by infrahepatic vena cava anastomosis. Alternatively, the donor vena cava can be anastomosed side to side with the recipient vena cava if it is left in situ during the recipient hepatectomy (piggyback technique). The operation then proceeds to the portal anastomosis. After all venous connections, the liver is reperfused with the suprahepatic vena cava temporarily occluded and the infrahepatic vena cava vented to allow washout of the hyperkalemic and adenosine-rich University of Wisconsin solution. The hepatic artery anastomosis is the final vascular step in the procedure.[4]

3. LUNG TRANSPLANTATION: correct answer a

Obliterative bronchiolitis is an inflammatory disorder of the small airways. Obliterative bronchiolitis has no predilection for sex or age, nor is it an indication for transplantation. Clinically, the patient may complain of dry or productive cough and dyspnea refractory to bronchodilators, along with generalized and progressive respiratory difficulty. The predominant functional abnormality is airflow obstruction, as evidenced by a serial decline in forced expiratory volume in 1 second. The histologic findings consist of dense fibrosis and scar tissue that obliterates the bronchial wall and lumen, along with bronchiectatic widening of the peripheral as well as the central bronchi. This fibrosis is irreversible, and there is no satisfactory treatment.[5]

4. TRANSPLANT IMMUNOLOGY: correct answer b

T lymphocytes play a key role in acute allograft rejection. Rejection may be mediated by T-helper lymphocytes through cytokines, which leads to the activation and proliferation of other cells, including B lymphocytes and macrophages. Acute allograft rejection may also occur through T-cytotoxic lymphocytes, which recognize and kill target cells.[6]

5. TRANSPLANT IMMUNOLOGY: correct answer e

MHC gene products are called human leukocyte antigens (HLAs). The MHC products are divided mainly into three different classes, which are expressed on different tissues and have different functions.

Class I MHC molecules are found on all nucleated cells. There are three different class I molecules: HLA-A, HLA-B, and HLA-C. The function of the class I MHC molecules is to act as the target for elimination of abnormal host cells, including infected cells with intracellular agents (viruses, intracellular bacteria, intracellular protozoal parasites, and intracellular fungi) and mutated or transformed cells (tumor cells).

Class II MHC molecules are found only on B lymphocytes, monocytes, macrophages, dendritic cells, Langerhans cells of the skin, activated endothelial cells, and activated human T cells. There are also three different class II molecules: HLA-DP, HLA-DQ, and HLA-DR. Class II molecules present exogenous (foreign) peptides to helper T lymphocytes.

HLA matching is not routinely performed before liver and cardiac transplantation. HLA matching is performed before transplantation of the kidney, pancreas, and lungs.[6]

6. TRANSPLANT IMMUNOLOGY: correct answer e

OKT3 is a murine monoclonal antibody that reacts with CD3 molecule on T lymphocytes, thereby blocking both the generation and function of the T cells in response to an antigenic challenge.

Cyclosporine is an inhibitor of the production and release of IL-2 and is metabolized through the cytochrome P450 enzyme system of the liver; its elimination is by urine, feces, and bile.

FK506 (tacrolimus) is also a potent inhibitor of IL-2. Cyclosporine and FK506 bind to intracellular proteins found in T cells known as *immunophilins.* This complex (immunophilin-FK506-cyclosporine) inhibits calcineurin. Calcineurin is an enzyme involved in the activation of genes responsible for the immune response. Inhibition of calcineurin blocks the production and release of IL-2.

Mycophenolate mofetil inhibits de novo purine synthesis. Both B and T lymphocytes depend on this metabolic pathway for proliferation and activation.

Steroids block IL-1, blunting the inflammatory response.

Rapamycin does not block IL-2 release and production; rapamycin blocks the IL-2 receptor, preventing cell proliferation and activation.[6]

7. TRANSPLANT IMMUNOLOGY: correct answer d

Rapamycin is a macrolide antibiotic derived from a fungus found in Rappanui (Easter Islands). The major side effects of rapamycin are hyperlipidemia and thrombocytopenia. Nephrotoxicity has not been demonstrated to be a side effect of rapamycin.

Cyclosporine is nephrotoxic and hepatotoxic and can cause hypertension, gingival hypertrophy, and hirsutism.

FK506 can lead to glucose intolerance, hyperkalemia, neurotoxicity, nephrotoxicity, and hepatotoxicity.

Mycophenolate mofetil is an antiproliferative agent that can cause diarrhea, leukopenia, and thrombocytopenia.

Reactions to OKT3 infusion are not uncommon and include fever, diarrhea, bronchospasm, pulmonary edema, and meningeal irritation.[6]

8. TRANSPLANT: correct answer a

Herpes simplex virus hepatitis, although uncommon, occurs early after solid organ transplantation, with a mean time of onset of 18 days. CMV hepatitis, which is much more frequent, has a peak time of onset of 35 days. Herpes simplex virus hepatitis is caused by human herpesvirus 1 (HHV-1) or HHV-2. The most common form of presentation of HHV-1 and HHV-2 is the eruption of small mucosal vesicles or ulcers. Dissemination to internal sites, including the esophagus, colon, and bladder, can occur, as can meningoencephalitis and ocular involvement with corneal and retinal infection. Active herpes simplex virus infection is diagnosed by culture of vesicular fluid, mucosal swabs, cerebrospinal fluid, or urine. Polymerase chain reaction testing can also be used; this technique is preferred for cerebrospinal fluid. A positive Tzanck smear signifies herpesvirus infection but is not specific for herpes simplex virus. Immunofluorescence staining with specific antisera is preferred. Acyclovir is the main drug used to treat herpes simplex virus infection.

Epstein-Barr virus is shed by 50% to 60% of patients after kidney transplantation. The major concern regarding Epstein-Barr virus infection is the development of post-transplantation lymphoproliferative disorder.

Seropositivity of CMV ranges from 40% to 80% in different populations. Without prophylaxis, half of the seropositive recipients of kidney transplantation from a CMV-seropositive donor experience CMV infection. Symptomatic CMV infection occurs in

10% of patients, independent of the initial donor serologic status.

"CMV syndrome," including fever, fatigue, leukopenia, and thrombocytopenia, occurs 1 to 6 months after infection. This syndrome may be accompanied by tissue-invasive symptoms such as pneumonitis, hepatitis, and gastritis. CMV infection of the kidney allograft is uncommon.

Diagnosis usually is confirmed by polymerase chain reaction. Prophylaxis in positive donor–negative recipients using intravenous ganciclovir during antilymphocyte therapy followed by 3 to 4 months of oral ganciclovir has been shown to decrease seroconversion and symptomatic CMV disease. Ganciclovir is also used in the treatment of CMV infections. Resistance to ganciclovir has been reported, but these strains are usually sensitive to foscarnet. CMV immune globulin is sometimes administered for severe CMV infection in addition to an antiviral agent, although controlled studies with kidney transplant recipients are lacking.

HHV-8 is the causative agent of Kaposi sarcoma. Limited and invasive Kaposi sarcoma can occur in transplant recipients. The limited form is characterized by the presence of violaceous skin nodules on the lower extremities. The invasive form is present mainly at the oropharynx, lungs, and GI tract. The mean time of onset is 21 months. The treatment consists of reduction or withdrawal of the immunosuppression.

BK poliovirus is a DNA virus that is trophic for the urinary tract. When infected, kidney transplant recipients present with hematuria, urinary obstruction, raised creatinine levels due to hemorrhagic cystitis, ureteral obstruction, or interstitial nephritis. Diagnosis can be confirmed by histologic examination, immunoperoxidase staining of biopsy tissue, detection of viral inclusions containing decoy cells via urine cytologic studies, or urine electron microscopy. No antiviral medication is available to treat polioviruses.[7]

9. TRANSPLANT: correct answer d

PTLDs are B-cell lymphomas. Four patterns of PTLD have been identified: uncomplicated infectious mononucleosis, benign polymorphic B-cell hyperplasia, polyclonal polymorphic B-cell lymphoma, and monoclonal polymorphic B-cell lymphoma.

Acute infection with Epstein-Barr virus most likely leads to an activation of the B cells with expansion of the lymphoid tissue and subsequent development of PTLD.

PTLD is responsible for 22% of tumors in transplant recipients, skin cancer being the most common post-transplantation cancer.

Up to 70% of patients with PTLD have extranodal involvement. Frequent sites are the central nervous system, GI tract, and allograft. The ileum and ascending colon are the sites most commonly involved in the GI tract.

Initial treatment consists of immunosuppression reduction or withdrawal and avoidance of antilymphocyte globulin therapy. Beyond reduction or discontinuation of immunosuppression, there is no consensus on the treatment of PTLD. Patients presenting early in the postoperative course, as well as patients with polymorphic disease, are more likely to experience a favorable course.[7]

10. TRANSPLANT: correct answer d

Lymphoceles are a frequent surgical complication after kidney transplantation: Some authors report an incidence of 18%. Clinical presentations typically are allograft dysfunction and hydronephrosis, ipsilateral lower limb edema secondary to lymphatic or venous compression, abdominal discomfort, or urinary frequency secondary to pressure on the bladder. The diagnosis is confirmed by ultrasound imaging or computed tomography. Although asymptomatic lymphoceles can be safely followed, intervention is indicated for symptomatic lymphoceles.

Arterial and venous graft thrombosis almost always leads to irreversible damage of the allograft. Warm ischemia time can be decreased, avoiding radiologic studies and operating as soon as possible if vascular thrombosis is considered likely.

The most common cause of a sudden drop in urinary output after kidney transplantation is a blood clot in the bladder or urethral catheter. Treatment consists only of flushing the Foley catheter.

Urinary leak usually occurs in the first weeks after transplantation. It is most often due to ureteral necrosis, which occurs after devascularization of the ureter during the donor nephrectomy. Other causes of urinary leak are technical error, bladder distention due to blood clot in the bladder, or infarction of the renal pelvis due to transection of the kidney pole arteries.[6, 8]

Quick Answers

1. D	6. E
2. A	7. D
3. A	8. A
4. B	9. D
5. E	10. A

REFERENCES

1. Doyle HR: Assessing risk in liver transplantation. Special reference to the significance of a positive cytotoxic cross match. Ann Surg 224:168–177, 1996.
2. Gruber S, Sutherland DER: Pancreas transplantation. Immunol Allergy Clin North Am 16:313–332, 1996.
3. Chen Y: Assessment of immunologic status of liver transplant recipients by peripheral blood mononuclear cells in response to stimulation by donor alloantigen. Ann Surg 230:242–250, 1999.
4. Sabiston D: The Biological Basis of Modern Surgical Practice, 15th ed. Philadelphia: WB Saunders, 1997, p 465.
5. Sabiston D: The Biological Basis of Modern Surgical Practice, 15th ed. Philadelphia: WB Saunders, 1997, pp 495–496.
6. Townsend CM, Sabiston DC, eds: Sabiston Textbook of Surgery: The Biological Basis of Modern Surgical Practice, 16th ed. Philadelphia: WB Saunders, 2001.
7. Smith SR, Butterly DW, Alexander BD, Greenberg A: Viral infections after renal transplantation. Am J Kidney Dis 37:659–676, 2001.
8. Hobart MG: Renal transplant complications. Minimally invasive management. Urol Clin North Am 27:787–798, 2000.

NOTES

Subspecialties

QUESTIONS

1. Regarding injuries to soft tissues, which of the following statements is correct?
   a. De Quervain tenosynovitis affects the first dorsal wrist compartment and involves the extensor pollicis brevis and abductor pollicis brevis.
   b. Dupuytren contracture is most common among manual laborers.
   c. The anterior cruciate ligament usually is injured after a varus force.
   d. The lateral meniscus is more frequently injured than the medial meniscus.
   e. The Thompson test is pathognomonic for Achilles tendon tear.

2. Regarding fractures, which of the following statements is incorrect?
   a. The treatment of a nondisplaced boxer's fracture is a plaster cast for 3 weeks.
   b. The body of the talus is an uncommon site of avascular necrosis.
   c. Colles fracture is a transverse fracture of the lower end of the radius with displacement of the distal fragment.
   d. Galeazzi fracture consists of a fracture of the distal radius with distal radioulnar joint dislocation.
   e. Monteggia fracture is a fracture of the upper third of the ulna with dislocation of the radial head.

3. Regarding soft tissue sarcomas, which is the most common histologic type found in the retroperitoneum?
   a. Malignant fibrous histiocytoma
   b. Leiomyosarcoma
   c. Liposarcoma
   d. Fibrosarcoma
   e. Rhabdomyosarcoma

4. Which is the clinical staging in a patient with Hodgkin disease who presents with fever, night sweats, weight loss, palpable left supraclavicular and left axillary nodes, and normal results with abdominal-pelvic computed tomography?
   a. IA
   b. IIA
   c. IIB
   d. IIIA
   e. IIIB
   f. IVA
   g. IVB

5. A 37-year-old female smoker presents with a 3-month history of a painless swelling near the right ear. There is no clinical regional nodal involvement, and intraoral examination results are normal. Fine-needle aspiration of the mass shows an acinic cell parotid cancer. Computed tomography reveals a 2.5-cm mass and no tumor invasion into the deep lobe of the parotid gland. The correct treatment for this patient should be
   a. Preoperative radiation therapy followed by a superficial parotidectomy
   b. Superficial parotidectomy only
   c. Total parotidectomy
   d. Total parotidectomy followed by chemotherapy

e. Superficial parotidectomy followed by radiation therapy

6. The left spermatic vein drains into the:
   a. Inferior vena cava
   b. Internal iliac vein
   c. Left pudendal vein
   d. Left renal vein
   e. Left inferior epigastric vein

7. In which of the following patients are intravenous steroids indicated as part of treatment?
   a. A 66-year-old woman with adult respiratory distress syndrome
   b. A 23-year-old man with closed head injury requiring intracranial pressure monitoring
   c. A 45-year-old woman with incomplete spinal cord injury
   d. A 9-year-old boy with partial-thickness burns of 33% of the total body surface
   e. A 41-year-old woman with fat embolism syndrome

8. Which of the following statements regarding the surgical management of a varicocele in adolescents is correct?
   a. Testicular growth arrest associated with varicocele is reversible, and catch-up growth of the testicle occurs after surgical correction.
   b. Prophylactic surgery is recommended in all adolescents with a varicocele.
   c. The left testicular vein drains into the ascending vena cava, inferior to the left renal vein.
   d. If the testicular artery is ligated during varicocele repair, the blood supply to the testicle becomes irreversibly compromised.
   e. Approximately 50% of men with varicocele are infertile.

9. A 69-year-old white man requests information about prostate cancer testing and risk factors. Which of the following is considered a risk factor for prostate cancer?
   a. Cigarette smoking
   b. Having a brother with prostate cancer
   c. Occupation
   d. Benign prostatic hypertrophy
   e. Sexual behavior

10. A 70-year-old woman presents with a 2-cm vulvar mass. A punch biopsy reveals a squamous carcinoma of the vulva with stromal invasion of less than 1 mm. The patient does not have any palpable nodes. What is the most appropriate treatment for this patient?
    a. Close observation only
    b. Wide local excision with a 2-cm gross margin
    c. Wide local excision with a 2-cm gross margin and ipsilateral groin dissection
    d. Radical vulvectomy with ipsilateral groin dissection
    e. Radical vulvectomy with bilateral groin dissection

11. What is the most appropriate treatment for a patient with a nonseminomatous germ cell tumor of the testicle and a 5-cm retroperitoneal mass?
    a. Orchiectomy only
    b. Orchiectomy and chemotherapy
    c. Orchiectomy, chemotherapy, and retroperitoneal lymph node dissection (RPLND)
    d. Orchiectomy, radiotherapy, and chemotherapy
    e. Orchiectomy and radiotherapy
    f. Orchiectomy, radiotherapy, and surgery (RPLND)
    g. Orchiectomy, radiotherapy, chemotherapy, and surgery (RPLND)

12. Regarding penile cancer, which one of the following is not true?
    a. Carcinoma in situ of the penis is called *erythroplasia of Queyrat* if it involves the glans penis, prepuce, or penile shaft.
    b. Circumcision has been well established as a prophylactic measure that virtually eliminates the occurrence of penile carcinoma.
    c. Clinically visceral metastases are not often detected.
    d. The prepuce is the site most commonly affected by penile cancer.
    e. Metastases to the regional femoral and iliac nodes are the earliest route of dissemination from penile carcinoma.

13. Regarding epithelial ovarian tumors, which one of the following statements is correct?
    a. Epithelial ovarian cancers usually secrete estrogen.
    b. CA-125 is elevated in approximately 80% of patients with epithelial ovarian cancer.
    c. Primary cytoreduction surgery is indicated only in the early stages of ovarian cancer.
    d. Mucinous cystadenocarcinoma is the most common epithelial ovarian tumor.
    e. After primary surgery, routine "second-look surgery" is considered the standard of care.

14. A 23-year-old white woman (P0,G0) presents to the emergency room with abdominal pain, fever, and a white blood cell count of 17,000/mm^3. Physical examination reveals abdominal tenderness and rebound in the right lower quadrant. Rectal and vaginal examination results are normal. Computed tomography of the abdomen and pelvis demonstrates an inflammatory mass on the right lower quadrant.

The patient is taken to the operating room with the preoperative diagnosis of acute appendicitis. During laparoscopy, you find the appendix to be normal and a right tubo-ovarian abscess with free pus in the pelvis. The most appropriate treatment for this patient is:

a. Appendectomy only
b. Oophorectomy only
c. Oophorectomy and salpingectomy
d. Oophorectomy, salpingectomy, and hysterectomy
e. Placement of pelvic drain and intravenous antibiotics

15. A 30-year-old black woman presents to the emergency room complaining of severe lower abdominal pain in the right lower quadrant and brisk vaginal bleeding. Her last menstrual period was 6 weeks earlier. A serum pregnancy test yields positive results, with a human chorionic gonadotropin titer of 2500 mIU/mL. Transvaginal ultrasonography demonstrates fluid in the pelvis, a normal appendix and ovaries, and an empty uterus. The most appropriate treatment for this patient is
    a. Bed rest and observation
    b. Linear salpingostomy
    c. Salpingostomy and oophorectomy
    d. Salpingectomy only
    e. Salpingectomy and oophorectomy

16. Regarding ovarian torsion, which one of the following statements is correct?
    a. Ovarian salvage is possible in half of cases.
    b. Most patients present with peritoneal signs.
    c. Initial radiographic work-up should include computed tomography of the abdomen and pelvis.

d. The laparoscopic approach is not adequate for treatment because of difficult visualization and exposure of the inflamed ovaries.
e. Untwisting of the adnexa is not associated with pulmonary embolism.

17. Regarding testicular torsion, which one of the following statements is correct?
    a. Most cases occur between the ages of 1 and 10 years.
    b. Reduction of the spermatic cord twist within 10 to 12 hours after initial presentation affords a good chance of salvaging the testis.
    c. The testis usually undergoes torsion in an inward or medial direction.
    d. Ultrasonographic evaluation is mandatory before surgery, even when clinical suspicion is high.
    e. Detorsion is accomplished through an inguinal incision.

18. Regarding prostatic cancer, which one of the following statements is correct?
    a. It accounts for the highest mortality among cancers in males.
    b. It is multifocal in more than 85% of cases.
    c. Transurethral resection of the prostate can be used as the primary therapy for certain types of prostate cancer.
    d. Positive pelvic nodes have minimal impact in the treatment of prostate cancer.
    e. Hormonal therapy and orchiectomy are indicated only for patients with disseminated metastatic disease.

19. Regarding renal carcinomas, which one of the following statements is correct?
    a. Half of patients present with the triad of hematuria, abdominal pain, and a palpable mass.

b. Radical nephroureterectomy is the treatment of choice for transitional cell cancers of the renal pelvis.
c. Adjuvant therapy with chemotherapy and radiotherapy results in a good outcome.
d. Nephrectomy with preservation of the adrenal gland is the surgical treatment of choice for renal cell carcinoma.
e. Half of patients with positive lymph node involvement survive 5 years.

20. Regarding bladder cancer, which one of the following statements is correct?
    a. The most common cancer of the bladder is squamous cell carcinoma.
    b. The treatment of choice for high-grade multifocal carcinoma in situ is radical cystectomy.
    c. Leukoplakia is not considered a premalignant lesion in the bladder.
    d. Carcinoma in situ carries a good prognosis (5-year survival exceeds 75%).
    e. At least a 5-cm surgical margin is required when performing partial cystectomy for solitary muscle infiltrative tumors.

21. A 35-year-old white woman sustained a 70% partial-thickness burn to her upper and lower extremities, chest, and back. You started her intravenous fluid resuscitation with Ringer's lactate using the Parkland formula. After 3 hours, her urinary output dropped and you noticed that her urine was dark and bloody. What is the most appropriate treatment for this patient?
    a. Give a 2-L bolus of Ringer's lactate.
    b. Give a 2-L bolus of normal saline.
    c. Give a 1-L bolus of hypertonic saline.
    d. Add 44 mEq of sodium bicarbonate/L of Ringer's lactate until the urine pH is >6.0.

e. Add 1 ampule of hydrochloric acid per liter of Ringer's lactate until the urine pH is <5.0.

22. Regarding nutrition of the burn patient, which one of the following statements is incorrect?
    a. Early enteral feedings decrease length of hospitalization.
    b. The Curreri formula is used to estimate the caloric needs of the burn patient.
    c. The greatest nitrogen loss is noticed mainly in the first 3 days after injury.
    d. The use of growth hormone has been reported to decrease the resting energy expenditure index.
    e. Burn wounds use glucose as the main source of energy.

23. Which one of the following is not a criterion for admitting a patient to a burn unit?
    a. An electrical burn
    b. A chemical burn
    c. Inhalation injury
    d. A 2% partial-thickness burn to the face in a patient with lupus and diabetes
    e. A 9% partial-thickness burn to the upper extremities and back

24. The most common cause of death of patients older than 65 years during the first 24 hours after a major burn injury is:
    a. Multisystem organ failure
    b. Sepsis
    c. Inhalation injury
    d. Cardiovascular collapse
    e. Associated trauma

25. A 30-year-old man sustained a chemical burn with hydrofluoric acid to his right forearm.

The most appropriate initial treatment for this patient is:

a. Normal saline irrigation or tap water irrigation only
b. 50% polyethylene glycol irrigation
c. Ethyl alcohol irrigation
d. Water-soaked pads followed by local application of petrolatum-based ointment
e. Water irrigation followed by topical application of calcium gel

26. A 70-kg 18-year-old man involved in a house fire sustained full-thickness burns to his entire back, right upper extremity, and posterior aspect of his right lower extremity. According to the Parkland formula, approximately how much fluid should this patient receive in the first 8 hours after injury?
    a. 5 L
    b. 6 L
    c. 7 L
    d. 8 L
    e. 9 L
    f. 10 L

27. Regarding electrical burns, which one of the following statements is incorrect?
    a. Direct current travels in one direction, and therefore an entrance and exit site may be evident.
    b. Lightning injuries are usually associated with deep burns.
    c. Electrical injuries are determined by the strength of the current and duration of exposure.
    d. Current is directly proportional to voltage and inversely proportional to resistance.
    e. The greatest resistance to electrical burns is found in the epidermis of the skin.

28. A 60-year-old white man comes into your office complaining of cough, hemoptysis, and weight loss. He has smoked one pack of cigarettes per day for 35 years. He has no other medical problems. A chest radiograph reveals a 4 × 4 cm central round mass in the lower lobe of the right lung. Computed tomography of the chest shows a central mass, 2 cm away the carina, with invasion of the visceral pleura, and questionable involvement of contralateral mediastinal nodes. Mediastinoscopy confirms the involvement of contralateral mediastinal nodes. The preoperative clinical staging, 5-year survival, and appropriate treatment for this patient are:
   a. I; 66%; right lower lobectomy
   b. II; 43%; right pneumonectomy
   c. IIIA; 23%; right middle and lower lobectomy
   d. IIIB; 5%; no surgery but chemotherapy and radiation
   e. IV; 5%; chemotherapy only

29. Regarding injuries to the lower extremities, which one of the following statements is incorrect?
   a. After a posterior knee dislocation, a study of the popliteal vessels is mandatory.
   b. A lateral tibial plateau fracture can occlude the anterior tibial artery and result in ischemic necrosis of the anterior compartment.
   c. Rupture of the anterior cruciate ligament is associated with damage of the medial collateral ligament.
   d. The lateral meniscus is injured more frequently than the medial meniscus.
   e. Distal tibiofibular ligament disruption generally requires surgical correction of the ankle.

30. Regarding fractures of the upper extremities, which one of the following statements is true?
    a. Open reduction of clavicle fractures usually has a better outcome than nonoperative treatment.
    b. Most fractures of the shaft of the humerus are treated by open reduction and fixation.
    c. Olecranon fractures rarely require open reduction and fixation.
    d. Monteggia fractures can be fixed by closed reduction of the radial head and internal fixation of the fractured ulna.
    e. Fractures of the shaft of the ulna and radius in children frequently require surgical intervention.

31. Diagnosis of a burn wound infection includes all of the following, except
    a. Black wound discoloration
    b. Violaceous wound margin
    c. Failure of a split-thickness skin graft to stick on the wound bed
    d. Adherent burn wound scar
    e. Greater than 10^5 microorganisms per gram of tissue on a burn wound biopsy specimen

ANSWERS

1. ACHILLES TENDON RUPTURE: correct answer e

The Thompson test, performed by squeezing the calf muscles to elicit plantar flexion with the patient in prone position, is pathognomonic of Achilles tendon tear when negative. De Quervain tenosynovitis affects the first dorsal wrist compartment and involves the extensor pollicis brevis and the abductor pollicis longus. The treatment involves splint, rest, steroid injection, and in some cases first-compartment release.

Dupuytren contracture, a contracture of the palmar aponeurosis, is thought to be inherited. The incidence is no higher in manual labor workers. Nonoperative management consists of exercise and local steroid injection. Partial or total palmar fascial excision is sometimes necessary.

Anterior cruciate ligament injury occurs after a valgus stress. The treatment varies with the patient's activity. In athletes, surgical repair is necessary. Conservative management is the treatment of choice in older patients.

The medial meniscus is more frequently injured than the lateral meniscus. Magnetic resonance imaging and arthroscopy are usually used for the diagnosis of a meniscus tear. When the tear is within the peripheral third of the meniscus and is less than 3 cm in length, repair should be performed.[1, 2]

2. TALUS AVASCULAR NECROSIS: correct answer b

The most common sites of avascular necrosis are the head of the femur, proximal half of the scaphoid bone, and body of the talus.

The treatment of a nondisplaced boxer's fracture, which consists of a fracture of the fourth or fifth metacarpal head, is a plaster cast for 3 weeks. Displaced boxer's fractures should undergo open reduction.

A Colles fracture is a transverse fracture of the lower end of the radius with displacement of the distal fragment. It occurs frequently in elderly women, and closed reduction is the initial treatment.

Open reduction should be performed if closed reduction fails.

A Galeazzi fracture is fracture of the distal radius with distal radioulnar joint dislocation. It usually requires open reduction and internal fixation.

A Monteggia fracture is fracture of the upper third of the ulna with dislocation of the radial head. Closed reduction of the radial head, if possible, and open reduction and internal fixation of the ulna constitute the treatment of choice.[1, 2]

3. SOFT TISSUE SARCOMAS: correct answer c

Liposarcoma is the most common sarcoma found in the retroperitoneum, followed by leiomyosarcoma. Malignant fibrous histiocytoma is the most common sarcoma of the extremities, followed by liposarcoma. The most common visceral sarcoma is the leiomyosarcoma. Fibrosarcoma, followed by malignant fibrous histiocytoma and liposarcoma, is the most common sarcoma on the trunk.

Treatment of sarcomas consists mainly of resection with a 2- to 3-cm margin. In tumors greater than 5 cm, external beam radiation or brachytherapy has been shown to decrease local recurrence. Chemotherapy is not beneficial in the treatment of soft tissue sarcomas.[1, 3, 4]

4. HODGKIN DISEASE: correct answer c

Hodgkin disease is a disorder primarily involving the lymphoid tissue. A distinct giant tumor cell known as Reed-Sternberg is essential in the diagnosis of Hodgkin disease. The staging is of great clinical importance and guides treatment. Staging involves a good history and physical examination, computed tomography of the abdomen and pelvis, chest radiography, and bone marrow biopsy. The Ann

Arbor stages for Hodgkin lymphoma are as follows (all stages are divided on the basis of the absence (A) or presence (B) of fever, weight loss, and night sweats):

Stage I: Involvement of a single lymph node region or involvement of a single extralymphatic organ or site (Ie)
Stage II: Involvement of two or more lymph node regions on the same side of the diaphragm alone (II) or with involvement of limited contiguous extralymphatic tissue (IIe)
Stage III: Involvement of lymph node regions on both sides of the diaphragm (III), which may include the spleen (IIIs) or limited contiguous extralymphatic organs or site (IIIe, IIIes), or both
Stage IV: Multiple or disseminated foci of involvement of one or more extralymphatic organs or tissues with or without lymphatic involvement

Four major histologic types have been defined: lymphocyte predominance, nodular sclerosis, mixed cellularity, and lymphocyte depletion. The most common type is nodular sclerosis followed by mixed cellularity and lymphocyte predominance. Nodular sclerosis is more common in women and young patients; involves the cervical, supraclavicular, and mediastinal nodes; and carries an excellent prognosis.

The indications for surgical staging in Hodgkin disease have decreased significantly. The advent of computed tomography and magnetic resonance imaging brought essential information regarding involvement of infradiaphragmatic organs. Currently, the indications for surgical staging are limited to stage I disease (disease apparently limited to one anatomic region); stage II disease demonstrates nodular sclerosis.

The staging procedure consists of a wedge liver biopsy, followed by splenectomy, removal of retroperitoneal and mesenteric nodes, and iliac marrow biopsy.[3, 5]

5. SALIVARY GLAND TUMORS: correct answer b

Acinic cell carcinoma accounts for 15% of parotid cancers. It has a low malignant potential with a 10-year survival rate of 70%. Superficial parotidectomy is the management of choice. Indications for postoperative radiation therapy include tumors greater than 4 cm, high-grade malignancies, recurrent or residual disease, and invasion of adjacent structures. Neck dissection is performed when nodes are clinically positive.[6, 7]

6. VASCULAR ANATOMY: correct answer d

On the right, the spermatic vein empties into the inferior vena cava below the right renal vein; on the left, the spermatic vein empties into the left renal vein.[6]

7. SPINAL CORD INJURY: correct answer c

Unlike traumatic brain injury, steroids have been shown to play an important role in improving outcome in patients with complete or incomplete spinal cord injury. Methylprednisolone should be administered as an intravenous bolus of 30 mg/kg, followed by a continuous infusion for at least 24 hours.[6]

8. VARICOCELE: correct answer a

Approximately 15% of all adult males have a varicocele. One third of all males evaluated for infertility have a varicocele, demonstrating the negative impact of varicoceles on testicular function. The arterial blood supply of the testis comes from the testicular artery, the deferential artery, and the cremasteric (or external spermatic) artery. Although the testicular artery is the major source of blood for the testis, there is collateral communication among these three arteries at the level of the testis; this collateral circulation can usually supply sufficient blood to the testis if the testicular artery is ligated during varicocele repair. The arteries supplying the testis course through the pampiniform plexus, and the arterial blood is cooled from the abdominal temperature (37°C) to testicular temperature (33°C) by countercurrent heat exchange with the veins of the pampiniform plexus. The right testicular vein joins the ascending vena cava, inferior to the right renal vein, whereas the left testicular vein joins the left renal vein. The deferential vein can provide venous return from the testicle after ligation of the varicocele.

Testicular growth arrest is reversible, and catch-up growth of the testicle occurs after surgical correction. The varicocele is the most common correctable cause of adult male infertility. Numerous studies have demonstrated an improvement in both semen quality and pregnancy rates after treatment. A varicocele repair in adolescents or pediatric patients with a varicocele is recommended for the following: a difference in testicular volume >2 mL as noted on serial ultrasonographic examinations, a decrease in testicular size of 2 standard deviations when compared with normal testicular growth curves, or scrotal pain. Prophylactic surgery in all adolescents with varicocele is not recommended.[8]

9. PROSTATE CANCER RISK FACTORS: correct answer b

Prostate cancer is the most common nondermatologic malignancy and the second leading cause of cancer mortality in men. It was estimated that in the year 2000, 1,800,400 new cases of prostate cancer would be diagnosed and that 31,900 men would die of the disease. Risk factors for prostate cancer include age, family history of prostate cancer, African American race and, possibly, dietary fat intake. More than 75% of all men in whom prostate cancer is diagnosed are older than 65 years. Men with a father or brother with prostate cancer are twice as likely to experience prostate cancer as men without affected relatives. The incidence of clinical prostate cancer is low in Asian men and higher in Scandinavian men. The age-adjusted incidence and mortality of prostate cancer are higher for African American men (234 and 56 per 100,000, respectively) than for white men (135 and 24 per 100,000, respectively). Other putative risk factors such as occupation, sexual behavior, infectious agents, vasectomy, cigarette smoking, and benign prostate conditions have not been demonstrated to alter the risk of prostate cancer.[9]

10. VULVAR CANCER: correct answer b

Wide local incision should be performed for stage I tumors if the lesion is microinvasive (< 1 mm invasion) with a 2-cm gross margin. Groin dissection should be performed for lesions that invade more than 1 mm. Bilateral groin dissection should be performed if the lesion is within 1 cm of the midline.

For stage II disease, radical vulvectomy with superficial and deep groin dissection is the treatment of choice.

Treatment is individualized in patients with stage III and stage IV disease. Options include surgery, radiation and chemotherapy, or a combination of treatment modalities (Table 14–1).

11. TESTICULAR CANCER: correct answer c

According to the M.D. Anderson Cancer Center staging system for testicular cancer, the treatment

TABLE 14–1

Staging for Carcinoma of the Vulva*

Stage Grouping

(Correlation of the FIGO, UICC, and AJCC nomenclatures)

AJCC/UICC				***FIGO***
Stage 0	Tis	N0	M0	
Stage I	T1	N0	M0	Stage I
Stage II	T2	N0	M0	Stage II
Stage III	T1	N1	M0	Stage III
	T2	N1	M0	
	T3	N0	M0	
	T3	N1	M0	
Stage IVA	T1	N2	M0	Stage IVA
	T2	N2	M0	
	T3	N2	M0	
	T4	Any N	M0	
Stage IVB	Any T	Any N	M1	Stage IVB

*From American Joint Committee on Cancer: Manual for Staging of Cancer, 4th ed. Philadelphia: JB Lippincott, 1992.

for stages IIB, C, and D to stage III consists of orchiectomy, systemic chemotherapy, and RPLND. RPLND is performed after initial chemotherapy to remove any residual disease and to determine the need for further therapy (Table 14–2).

12. PENILE CANCERS: correct answer d

Approximately 50% of penile cancers involve the penile glans, 21% the prepuce, 9% both prepuce and glans, 6% the coronal sulcus, and 2% the shaft of the penis. Carcinoma in situ of the penis is also

TABLE 14–2

M.D. Anderson Cancer Center Staging Systems for Testicular Cancer

Stage	*Description*	*Treatment*
Seminoma		
I	Confined to testicle	Orchiectomy + radiation
IIA	Retroperitoneal disease only, mass <10 cm	Orchiectomy + radiation
IIB	Retroperitoneal disease only, mass >10 cm	Chemotherapy
IIIA	Subdiaphragmatic nodal disease	Chemotherapy*
IIIB	Visceral disease	Chemotherapy*
Nonseminomatous Germ Cell Tumor		
I	Confined to the testicle	Orchiectomy + RPLND†
IIA	Negative clinical, positive surgical, RPLND or elevated markers post orchiectomy	Orchiectomy + RPLND

IIB	RPLND mass <2 cm	Orchiectomy + chemotherapy + RPLND‡
IIC	RPLND mass <5 cm	Orchiectomy + chemotherapy + RPLND‡
IID	RPLND mass <10 cm	Orchiectomy + chemotherapy + RPLND‡
IIIA	Supraclavicular node disease	Individualized treatment§
IIIB1	Elevated markers post RPLND	Individualized treatment§
IIIB2	Pulmonary disease	Individualized treatment§
IIIB3	Advanced abdominal disease (mass >10 cm)	Individualized treatment§
IIIB4	Visceral disease other than lung	Individualized treatment§
IIIB5	β-human chorionic gonadotropin >50,000 ± IIIB2, IIIB4	Individualized treatment§

*Surgery is indicated when lymphatic disease does not respond to chemotherapy.
†Treatment is controversial: orchiectomy only, or orchiectomy + RPLND.
‡Primary systemic chemotherapy is the treatment of choice.
§Primary systemic chemotherapy is the treatment of choice. RPLND is used to remove residual lymphatic disease.
RPLND, retroperitoneal lymph node dissection.

called *erythroplasia of Queyrat* if it involves the glans, penis, prepuce, or penile shaft, and is called *Bowen disease* if it involves other regions of the penis. Treatment for these lesions, when small, can be achieved through local excision, radiation therapy, laser therapy, and topical 5-fluorouracil, 5%.

Penile cancer in circumcised patients is extremely rare. Indeed, the appearance of penile tumors in uncircumcised men has been attributed to chronic irritation of smegma, a byproduct of bacterial action on desquamated cells that are within the prepuce.

Visceral metastases to the lung, liver, bone, or brain are uncommon and occur in 1% to 10% of cases. Metastases to the regional femoral and iliac nodes are the earliest routes of dissemination from penile carcinoma.

The strongest prognostic indicator for survival continues to be the presence or absence of nodal metastases; 20% to 50% of patients with clinically palpable adenopathy have histologically proven inguinal node metastases and should be treated with inguinal lymphadenectomy.

The gold standard of treatment of penile cancer is partial or total penectomy. At least a 2-cm margin is necessary on the partial penectomies to avoid local recurrence. If the tumor involves the shaft and a 2-cm margin is not possible, total penectomy with perineal urethrostomy is the procedure of choice. Laser therapy has been used to treat many benign and premalignant penile lesions as well as stage Tis, Ta, T1, and some T2 penile cancers. Potential advantages of laser therapy in penile cancer are destruction of the lesion with preservation of normal structure and function. Currently, four types of lasers are used in the treatment of penile lesions: CO_2, Nd:YAG, argon, and potassium titanyl phosphate.[10]

13. OVARIAN CANCER: correct answer b

CA-125 is elevated in approximately 80% of patients with epithelial ovarian cancers. CA-125 can be used to follow patients with ovarian cancer after treatment has been established. The most common histologic type of ovarian cancer is serous cystadenocarcinoma, accounting for approximately 46% of cases, followed by mucinous (36%), endometrioid (8%), clear cell (3%), and transitional (2%).

The initial step in the treatment of ovarian cancer is surgical cytoreduction, which includes total abdominal hysterectomy, bilateral salpingo-oophorectomy, infracolic omentectomy with or without appendectomy, and selective pelvic and para-aortic lymph node sampling. Primary cytoreduction is a key component of treatment, especially in advanced cases. Routine second-look surgery is no longer considered the standard of care.[11]

14. OBSTETRICS-GYNECOLOGY: correct answer e

Pelvic inflammatory disease after misdiagnosis of appendicitis requires no further intervention, unless gross purulent contamination is present, in which case pelvic drains should be inserted. The initial treatment for pelvic inflammatory disease consists of antibiotic therapy. If symptoms are not severe, outpatient treatment with oral antibiotics is sufficient. Surgery is not indicated unless medical therapy fails. Patients with rupture of a pelvic abscess require intravenous antibiotics and drainage, which can be percutaneous. If there is no improvement after antibiotic therapy and drainage, an exploratory laparotomy, oophorectomy, salpingectomy, and total hysterectomy should be considered.[1]

15. OBSTETRICS-GYNECOLOGY: correct answer d

Salpingectomy is the treatment of choice in patients with ruptured tubal pregnancy. Linear salpingostomy may be indicated when the fallopian tubes are not severely damaged. Oophorectomy is not indicated in cases of ectopic pregnancy. In unruptured ectopic pregnancy, linear salpingostomy is the procedure of choice. After surgery, serial human chorionic gonadotropin levels should be followed to zero if the fallopian tube is left in place.

16. OVARIAN TORSION: correct answer e

Inclusion in the differential diagnosis and a high index of suspicion are key to the diagnosis of ovarian torsion. Most patients present with sudden onset of moderate to severe crampy or sharp lower abdominal pain, with radiation to the flank or groin associated with nausea and vomiting. On physical examination, patients have mild to moderate abdominal tenderness and a palpable mass on vaginal examination. Infrequently, patients present with peritoneal signs. Initial radiologic evaluation should begin with Doppler ultrasonography of the ovaries. In the great majority of cases, size, flow, and associated ovarian pathology can be evaluated ultrasonically.

Laparoscopy or open abdominal explorations are adequate to evaluate and treat ovarian torsion. Ovarian salvage through ovarian detorsion is only possible in a few cases. Most patients undergo unilateral oophorectomy and salpingectomy because of ischemic changes of the ovaries and fallopian tubes.

Ovarian cysts are frequently associated with ovarian torsion. Also, previous tubal ligation is commonly part of the medical history of patients who experience ovarian torsion. Malignancy is rarely associated with ovarian torsion but has been reported.[12]

17. TESTICULAR TORSION: Correct answer c

The testicle usually undergoes torsion in an inward or medial direction. When manual detorsion is attempted, the testis should be turned two or three rotations in a lateral-outward direction. Manual detorsion is not a temporary solution and should not delay definitive surgical correction.

Most cases of testicular torsion occur between the ages of 12 and 18 years, but this entity also often occurs in infants. Reduction of the spermatic twist within 6 hours of the initial onset of symptoms affords a good chance of salvaging the testis. Ultrasonographic imaging is not mandatory in the evaluation of testicular torsion. If clinical suspicion is high, surgical exploration should be performed immediately.

Detorsion is performed through a scrotal incision. The testis undergoes detorsion and is assessed for viability. If it remains dark, the testis is probably nonviable. Meanwhile, as one is waiting to reassess viability, contralateral orchiopexy should be performed. If the testis is nonviable, orchiectomy is indicated.[13]

18. PROSTATE CANCER: correct answer b

Prostate cancer is multifocal in more than 85% of cases. Most tumors are also peripherally located. With palpable tumors, the final surgical pathology specimen shows that more than 70% of patients have a contralateral malignancy.

Prostate cancer is the most common malignancy in the male population. The malignancy that kills most Americans (men and women) is lung cancer. Physical examination, including rectal digital examination in combination with prostate-specific antigen levels and transrectal ultrasonography, followed by transrectal prostatic biopsy, reliably diagnoses prostate cancer. The use of prostate-specific antigen without digital rectal examination is not recommended because 25% of men with prostate cancer have prostate-specific antigen levels less than 4.0 ng/mL. Positive pelvic nodes are an important prognostic factor, precluding radical prostatectomy and requiring androgen ablation as treatment. Pelvic nodes are positive in 5% to 7% of patients. Hormonal therapy is indicated for patients with positive pelvic nodes, patients with disseminated metastatic disease, and older patients who are not suitable for surgery or are not going to benefit from surgical therapy in the long term. Radical prostatectomy should be reserved for men who are likely to be cured and will live long enough to benefit from the cure.[13]

19. UROLOGY: correct answer b

Radical nephroureterectomy is the treatment of choice for transitional cell cancers of the renal pelvis. These tumors are multifocal and tend to present not only in the pelvis but also in the ureter. Only 10% of patients present with the triad of hematuria, abdominal pain, and a palpable mass. The most common complaint of patients with renal cell carcinoma is hematuria. Adjuvant chemotherapy and radiotherapy has been shown to have minimal effect on patients with renal cell carcinoma and does not change the progression of the disease. Long-term survival can be achieved only through surgical resection. Radical nephrectomy, which includes resection of the Gerota fascia and perirenal fat, kidney, and adrenal gland, is considered the standard surgical therapy for patients with renal cell carcinoma. Long-term survival is dismal if lymph nodes are involved. The 5-year survival rate in patients with positive lymph nodes varies between 0% and 30%.[13]

20. UROLOGY: correct answer b

The diagnosis of carcinoma in situ usually portends a poor outcome. Carcinoma in situ is most often associated with high-grade neoplasia and carries a bad prognosis.

More than 90% of bladder malignancies are transitional cell tumors. Squamous cell carcinomas account for 5%. In Egypt, more than 75% of bladder cancers are squamous cell carcinoma. About 80% of those are associated with chronic infection with *Schistosoma haematobium.*

Leukoplakia is considered a premalignant lesion and can progress to invasive bladder carcinoma.

The treatment of bladder cancer depends on the invasiveness of the tumor. Bladder cancers can be detected while still confined to the mucosa or lamina propria, and they can be treated by endoscopic resection with or without intravesical therapy (chemotherapy or bacille Calmette-Guérin). Partial cystectomy is considered for selected cases in which a single tumor is present and a 2-cm margin of resection can be obtained. Radical cystectomy is considered for tumors that invade the bladder muscularis and for high-grade, anaplastic, multifocal carcinoma in situ.[13]

21. BURNS: correct answer d

Presence of myoglobin in the urine due to rhabdomyolysis in patients with extensive burns is common, especially in patients with an electrical burn injury.

The treatment consists of alkalinization of the urine, adding 44 mEq of sodium bicarbonate/L of Ringer's lactate, until the urine pH is >6.0. Alkalinization of the urine prevents precipitation of hemoglobin in the renal tubules, avoiding acute renal failure.[14]

22. BURNS: correct answer c

The main source of energy for burn wounds is glucose.

Some reports have shown that growth hormone improves the nutritional status and decreases the resting energy expenditure index.

Early enteral feedings decrease the level of catabolic hormones, decreasing the hypermetabolic state. They also maintain gut integrity, decrease episodes of diarrhea, and decrease the length of hospital stay.

The Curreri formula can be used along with indirect calorimetry to estimate the caloric needs of a burn patient. The Curreri formula is based on weight (kg) and the extent of the burn. In adults aged 16 to 59 years, the formula is:

$$Cf = 25 \text{ kcal/kg} + 40 \text{ cal} \times \% \text{ burn}$$

In adults older than 59 years:

$$Cf = 20 \text{ kcal/kg} + 65 \text{ cal} \times \% \text{ burn}$$

The greatest nitrogen loss usually occurs between the 5th and 10th postburn days.[14]

23. BURNS: correct answer e

Burn injuries that should be referred to a burn center include all of the following:

Partial-thickness burn >10% total body surface area
Burns that involve face, hands, feet, genitalia, perineum, or major joints
Third-degree burns in any age group
Electrical burns, including those caused by lightning

Chemical burns
Inhalation injury
Burn injury in patients with preexisting medical disorders that could complicate management, prolong recovery, or affect mortality
Any patient with burns and concomitant trauma (such as fracture) in which the burn injury poses the greatest risk of morbidity and mortality; in such cases, if trauma poses the greater immediate risk, the patient may be initially stabilized in a trauma center before being transferred to the burn center; physician judgment is necessary in such situations and should be in concert with the regional medical control plan and triage protocols
Burned children in hospitals without qualified personnel or equipment for the care of children
Burn injury in patients who will require special social, emotional, or long-term rehabilitative intervention[14]

24. BURNS: correct answer d

The three most important prognostic variables in predicting whether patients will survive the burn injury are the patient's age, the size and depth of the burn injury, and the presence or absence of an inhalation injury. At present, the mean published burn size associated with a 50% mortality rate ranges from 65% to 75% of the total body surface area.

Patients older than 65 years are most likely to succumb to their injury in the first 24 hours, especially when the burn wounds exceed 60% of the total body surface area. The two major causes of early death are cardiovascular collapse and multiple organ failure. Multiple organ failure is most likely in patients younger than 40 years, and cardiovascular collapse occurs in patients older than 65 years as a cause of early death.[15]

25. BURNS: correct answer e

After hydrofluoric acid exposure, the wound should be vigorously irrigated with water, followed by the topical application of calcium gel to neutralize the fluoride (one ampule of calcium gluconate and 100 g of lubricating jelly). Patients with persistent pain might require intra-arterial administration of calcium.

Plain sterile water is usually used to irrigate chemical burns.

On chemical burns caused by phenol, an acidic alcohol with poor water solubility, irrigation with water followed by cleansing with 50% polyethylene glycol or ethyl alcohol is adequate.

Hot tar burns can also be considered chemical burns. Treatment consists of cooling the molten material with cold water. After the burn wound is cooled, adherent tar can be covered with a petrolatum-based ointment, which promotes emulsification of the tar.[14]

26. BURNS: correct answer a

Adequate fluid resuscitation plays a key role in the care of the burn patient. Many formulas have been used to resuscitate burn patients, but the Parkland formula is by far the most common. This formula uses the weight of the patient and the extent of partial- or full-thickness burns multiplied by 4 to estimate the amount of fluids that burn patients will need for the first 24 hours:

$$PF = 4 \times \text{weight in kg} \times \%\ \text{burn}$$

Half of the calculated amount is given in the first 8 hours and the other half in the subsequent 16 hours.[14]

27. BURNS: correct answer b

Lightning injuries usually are associated with superficial skin and soft tissue injuries. Lightning injuries are associated with a 30% mortality rate due to their potential to cause significant cardiac and neurologic damage. Lightning is direct current with a voltage that may exceed 200,000 volts. Direct current travels in one direction, so exit and entrance sites may be visible. With alternating current, the electricity flows back and forth from the power source to the anatomic contact point on the patient; therefore, exit or entrance wounds might not be visible.

The current and duration of exposure determine the extent of an electrical injury. The Ohm law states that $I = V/R$ where I is current, V is voltage, and R is resistance.

The skin is the organ most resistant to electrical current. The epidermis has the greatest resistance.[14]

28. LUNG CANCER: correct answer d

TNM staging for non–small cell cancer is used as a guideline for treatment and prognosis. In the TNM system, T describes the tumor itself as follows: *TX,* occult carcinoma; *T1,* tumor <3 cm, surrounded by lung or visceral pleura but not proximal to a lobar bronchus; *T2,* tumor >3 cm or with involvement of main bronchus at least 2 cm distal to the carina, or with visceral pleura involvement, or associated with atelectasis, obstructive pneumonitis, extending to the hilar region, but not involving the entire lung; *T3,* tumor invading chest wall, diaphragm, mediastinal pleura, or parietal pericardium, or tumor in the main bronchus within 2 cm of, but not invading, carina, or atelectasis of obstructive pneumonitis of the entire lung; *T4,* tumor invading mediastinum, heart, great vessels, trachea, esophagus, vertebral body, or carina, or ipsilateral malignant effusion.

N represents the involvement of the nodes: *N0,* no regional lymph node metastases; *N1,* metastases to ipsilateral peribronchial or hilar nodes; *N2,* metastases to ipsilateral mediastinal or subcarinal nodes; *N3,* metastases to contralateral mediastinal or hilar nodes or to any scalene or supraclavicular nodes.

M describes the absence or presence of metastases: *M0,* no distant metastases; *M1,* distant metastases.

The following stage grouping, according the American Joint Committee on Cancer and the International Union Against Cancer (AJCC/UICC), predicts the 5-year survival for non–small cell carcinoma according to the stage:

Stage I	66.7%
Stage II	43%
Stage IIIA	22%
Stage IIIB	5%
Stage IV	5%

Mediastinoscopy is a useful tool when the diagnosis of contralateral node involvement is uncertain. Patients with stage IIIB disease are not candidates for surgery. Radiation therapy and combination chemotherapy, which includes cisplatin and vinca alkaloids or cisplatin and etoposide, have been reported to yield response rates of 20% to 50%.[1]

29. ORTHOPEDICS: correct answer d

The medial meniscus is injured at least four times more often than the lateral meniscus. Magnetic resonance imaging can be used for diagnosis of this injury. Arthroscopy can be used for the diagnosis and treatment of these injuries.

A study of the popliteal vessels is mandatory after a posterior knee dislocation. Injury of the popliteal vessels can be present in up to 40% of cases, and delay in diagnosis and repair has led to amputation rates as high as 85%.

A lateral tibial plateau fracture can present with anterior compartment leg necrosis due to thrombosis of the anterior tibial artery. Neurovascular injury occurs in 50% of cases.

Usual indications for surgical repair of an ankle fracture are bimalleolar fracture, trimalleolar fracture, and tibiofibular ligament disruption.[2]

30. ORTHOPEDICS: correct answer d

The treatment of a Monteggia fracture (dislocation of the head of the radius and fracture of the proximal ulna) remains controversial. Most authors recommend closed reduction of the radial head and internal fixation of the fractured ulna. When closed reduction of the radial head is not possible, open reduction should be performed.

Most fractures of the clavicle can be treated conservatively. Nonunion occurs in less than 1% of patients, whereas it occurs in 4% of patients who undergo surgery.

Most fractures of the shaft of the humerus can be treated nonoperatively. Nonsurgical treatment results in a higher incidence of union and fewer complications than does open reduction and internal fixation. Conversely, in fractures of the olecranon in adults, when the fragments are separated, open reduction and internal fixation are necessary.

Fractures of the radius and ulna most likely do not require open reduction in children. Because of the high impact and subsequent displacement of the radius and ulna, this fracture is treated with open reduction and fixation in adults.[2]

31. BURN WOUND INFECTION: correct answer d

A black wound, wound discoloration, violaceous and edematous wound borders, conversion from a partial-thickness to a full-thickness burn wound, and failure of a split-thickness graft to adhere to the wound bed are all indications of an infected burn wound. Infection can be confirmed with a quantitative burn wound biopsy, which will show a count greater than 10^5 microorganisms per gram of tissue.[1]

Quick Answers

1. E	9. B	17. C	25. E
2. B	10. B	18. B	26. A
3. C	11. C	19. B	27. B
4. C	12. D	20. B	28. D
5. B	13. B	21. D	29. D
6. D	14. E	22. C	30. D
7. C	15. D	23. E	31. D
8. A	16. E	24. D	

REFERENCES

1. Townsend CM, Sabiston DC, eds: Sabiston Textbook of Surgery: The Biological Basis of Modern Surgical Practice, 16th ed. Philadelphia: WB Saunders, 2001.
2. Canale ST: Campbell's Operative Orthopedics, 9th ed. St. Louis: CV Mosby, 1998.
3. Schwartz SI: Principles of Surgery, 7th ed. New York: McGraw-Hill, 1999.
4. Cotran RS: Robbins Pathologic Basis of Disease, 6th ed. Philadelphia: WB Saunders, 1999.
5. Robbins SL: Pathologic Basis of Disease, 5th ed. Philadelphia: WB Saunders, 1994.
6. Sabiston D: The Biological Basis of Modern Surgical Practice, 15th ed. Philadelphia: WB Saunders, 1997, pp 1322–1324.

7. Nyhus L, Baker R, Fischer J: Mastery of Surgery, 3rd ed. Boston: Little, Brown, 1997, pp 302–305.
8. Skoog S, Roberts KP, Goldstein M, Pryor JL: The adolescent varicocele: what's new with an old problem in young patients? Pediatrics 100:112–122, 1997.
9. Liang B: Early detection and treatment of prostate cancer. Hosp Phys 37:54–67, 2000.
10. Ryan KJ: Kistner's Gynecology & Women's Health, 7th ed. St. Louis: CV Mosby, 1999.
11. Feig BW, Berger DH, Fuhrman GM: The M.D. Anderson Surgical Oncology Handbook, 2nd ed. Philadelphia: Lippincott Williams & Wilkins, 1999.
12. Houry D, Abbott J: Ovarian torsion: a fifteen-year review. Ann Emerg Med 38:156–159, 2001.
13. Walsh PC: Campbell's Urology, 7th ed. Philadelphia: WB Saunders, 1998.
14. Advanced burn life support course, provider's manual. American Burn Association, Chicago, 2001.
15. Herndon DN: Total Burn Care, 3rd ed. Philadelphia: WB Saunders, 2000.

NOTES

PART THREE

High-Yield Facts

David Brandli, M.D.

Patrick Connolly, M.D.

Virgilio George, M.D.

William Hoffman, M.D.

Anesthesia for the General Surgeon

Virgilio George, M.D.

Causes of Hypoxemia

Low inspired oxygen concentration
Hypoventilation
Shunt
Ventilation-perfusion (V/Q) inequality or mismatch

Causes of Hypercarbia

Hypoventilation, including muscle paralysis, inadequate ventilation, inhalational anesthetics, and opiates

Effects of Inhalational Anesthetics on Ventilation

They attenuate the ventilatory response to hypercarbia and hypoxemia. Delivery of anesthetic gases results in dose-dependent depression of ventilation mediated directly through medullary centers and indirectly through effects on intercostal muscle function.

How Does Positive End-Expiratory Pressure (PEEP) Work?

PEEP increases oxygenation by maximizing the ventilation-perfusion relationship in the lung. PEEP maximizes the functional residual capacity, keeping lung volumes greater than closing capacity, therefore maintaining open and functional airways.

What Adverse Effects Could the Addition of PEEP Produce?

Decreased venous return
Decreased cardiac output
Hypotension
Worsening hypoxia
Barotrauma (pneumothorax)
Increased intracranial pressure
Decreased urine output

What Are the Causes of a Sudden Decrease in End-Tidal Carbon Dioxide in an Anesthetized Patient?

Low cardiac output
Pulmonary embolism
Venous air embolism
Circuit leak or disconnection
Extubation
Obstruction of the airway or sampling tubing
Cardiac arrest

Indications for Endotracheal Intubation

Profound disturbances in consciousness with inability to protect the airway
Tracheobronchial toilet
Severe pulmonary and multisystem injury associated with respiratory failure (severe sepsis, airway obstruction, hypoxemia, and hypercarbia of various causes)

Objective Measures that Suggest the Need for Intubation

Respiratory rate >35 breaths per minute
Vital capacity <15 mL/kg in adults and 10 mL/kg in children
Inability to generate a negative inspiratory force of 20 mmHg
Pao_2 <70 mmHg on 40% oxygen
A-a gradient >350 mmHg on 100% oxygen
$Paco_2$ >55 mmHg (except in chronic retainers)
Dead space (Vd/Vt) >0.6

Rapid Sequence Induction (RSI)

The usual RSI begins with preoxygenation with 100% oxygen. Induction agents that are often used in hemodynamically unstable patients include ketamine and etomidate. Reduced doses are used in trauma patients because of contracted blood volume. The muscle relaxant of choice is succinylcholine, which has the faster onset of paralysis for intubation. Before the anesthetic and succinylcholine are administered, pressure is applied firmly over the cricoid ring (Sellick maneuver) to prevent regurgitation of gastric contents. The patient is intubated as soon as adequate muscle relaxation is achieved (approximately 45 to 60 seconds).

What Are the Most Common Neuromuscular Blocking Agents Used?

Depolarizing
Succinylcholine (Sch)
Nondepolarizing
Mivacurium

Rocuronium
Vecuronium
Atracurium
Cisatracurium
Pancuronium

What Are the Adverse Effects of Succinylcholine?

Its duration of action can be prolonged unpredictably in the presence of pseudocholinesterase deficiency (in liver disease, pregnancy, malnutrition, and malignancies).

Succinylcholine stimulates all cholinergic receptors, and all types of arrhythmias can occur, especially bradycardia.

Hyperkalemia can occur when a proliferation of extrajunctional receptors is present.

Succinylcholine can trigger malignant hyperthermia.

Succinylcholine increases intracranial pressure (ICP) and intraocular pressure.

When Is Succinylcholine Contraindicated?

From about 24 hours after a burn injury until the burn has healed, succinylcholine may cause hyperkalemia because of proliferation of extrajunctional neuromuscular receptors.

Muscular dystrophies

Prolonged immobility

Spinal cord injury

Upper and lower motor neuron disease

Closed head injury

What Is MAC?

Minimal alveolar concentration: the concentration at 1 atmosphere that abolishes motor response to a painful stimulus (surgical incision) in 50% of patients

Why Can Nitrous Oxide Be Dangerous?

It is 20 times more soluble than nitrogen. Thus, nitrous oxide can diffuse 20 times faster into closed spaces than it can be removed, resulting in expansion of pneumothorax, bowel gas, or air embolism or in increased pressures within noncompliant cavities such as the cranium or middle ear.

Which Anesthetic Gas Is Associated with the Greatest Frequency of Cardiac Dysrhythmias?

Halothane

Which Anesthetic Gas Has Been Shown to Be Teratogenic in Animals?

Nitrous oxide, which has been shown to increase skeletal abnormalities; the mechanism is thought to be related to inhibition of methionine synthesis; it may be prudent to limit use of this agent in pregnant women.

Thiopental Sodium (Pentothal)

It causes dose-dependent central nervous system (CNS) depression, with hypnosis and amnesia, and confers seizure protection because it reduces the functional activity of the brain and the brain metabolism.

The usual intravenous (IV) induction dose of 3 to 5 mg/kg produces a loss of consciousness within 15 seconds and recovery within 5 to 10 minutes. It is 99% metabolized by the liver.

Methohexital (Brevital)

Causes dose-dependent CNS depression with hypnosis and amnesia, but does not confer seizure protection.

The usual IV induction dose is 1 to 2 mg/kg, with loss of consciousness and a recovery rate similar to those of thiopental. However, the clearance rate is faster. Full recovery for CNS effects is significantly more rapid than with thiopental.

Propofol (Diprivan)

IV sedative hypnotic agent used for induction and maintenance of anesthesia as well as sedation; it is formulated in a white soybean oil, egg yolk, and lecithin emulsion (essential intralipid 10%).

The usual IV induction dose of 2 to 2.5 mg/kg produces loss of consciousness in less than 1 minute and lasts for 4 to 6 minutes.

During induction, rapid arterial and venous vasodilation and a mild negative inotropic effect cause a decrease in blood pressure of 20% to 30%. This decrease is usually most profound in patients who are hypovolemic and may be reduced by a slow rate of infusion and pre-induction volume loading.

Etomidate (Amidate)

It is structurally unrelated to any of the other IV anesthetic agents. The induction dose of 0.2 to 0.4 mg/kg IV provides rapid loss of consciousness, which lasts 3 to 12 minutes. The duration of CNS depression is dose dependent. Myoclonus during induction may occur secondary to disinhibition of subcortical neuronal activity. The incidence of nausea and vomiting is fairly high.

Ketamine (Ketalar)

Ketamine is a phencyclidine derivative. It produces rapid CNS depression with hypnosis (within 30 seconds), sedation, amnesia, and analgesia. The induction doses are 1 to 2 mg/kg IV, with effects lasting 5 to 10 minutes, or 10 mg/kg IM, which acts in 3 to 5 minutes. Clearance depends on hepatic blood flow.

Ketamine is unique in that it stimulates the cardiovascular system, increasing heart rate, blood pressure, and cardiac output; such effects are not dose dependent. In addition, ketamine provides bronchial smooth muscle relaxation.

Ketamine has a high incidence of disturbing “bad trips” or emergence delirium, described as out-of-body sensation and illusion. Salivary gland secretion is increased.

Which IV Induction Drug Increases ICP?

Ketamine increases cerebral blood flow, ICP, and cerebral metabolism and is contraindicated in patients with elevated intracranial pressure.

Etomidate, thiopental, propofol, and fentanyl all reduce ICP secondary to a decrease in cerebral blood flow and cerebral metabolic consumption of oxygen.

Which Intravenous Anesthetics Are Recommended for Use in Trauma or Other Hypovolemic Cases?

Ketamine is recommended for patients who are acutely hypovolemic because of its sympathomimetic effect on increasing heart rate and peripheral vasoconstriction.

Etomidate also may be used as an induction agent in trauma because of its cardiovascular stability.

Propofol may be used in hemodynamically stable patients who present with possible head trauma.

What Are the Side Effects of Benzodiazepines?

Midazolam (Versed), diazepam (Valium), and lorazepam (Ativan) are most commonly used.

Midazolam is water-soluble, with sedative hypnotic and amnestic (antegrade) properties. Midazolam causes the least venous irritation of all benzodiazepines.

The major side effects of diazepam and lorazepam are venous irritation and thrombophlebitis secondary to the presence of organic solvents; both drugs are water-insoluble.

Prolonged amnesia, sedation, and rare cases of significant respiratory depression may occur with all of these agents.

What Are the Clinical Effects of Benzodiazepines?

Benzodiapines result in anxiolysis, sedation, amnesia, suppression of seizure activity, and (in high doses) unconsciousness and respiratory depression. The effects are dose dependent. Benzodiazepines are not analgesics.

How Can the Effect of Benzodiazepines Be Reversed?

Flumazenil is a competitive antagonist and reverses all the effects of benzodiazepines. Flumazenil is given in increments of 0.2 mg IV until respiratory depression or sedation is reversed.

The side effect is the need for resedation because of the short half-life when compared with the elimination half-life of benzodiazepines. Resedation can be accomplished with repeated doses or continuous infusion of 0.5 to 1.0 μg/kg/min.

What Opioid Receptor Is Responsible for Respiratory Depression?

μ : Morphine

μ_2: Respiratory depression, bradycardia, physical dependence, euphoria, and ileus

κ : Analgesia, sedation, dysphoria, and psychomimetic effects

μ_1: Analgesia

δ : Modulates activity at the μ receptor

σ : Dysphoria, hypertonia, tachycardia, tachypnea, and mydriasis

What Is the Mechanism of Action of Neuroaxial Opioids?

Opioids are injected into the epidural or intrathecal space. They bind to receptors in the dorsal horn of the spinal cord, more specifically in the substantia gelatinosa. This is the area that processes afferent pain information and contains opioid receptors.

What Are the Adverse Effects of Neuroaxial Opioids?

Pruritus
Nausea and vomiting
Urinary retention
Ventilatory depression

Compared with Parenteral Opioids, What Are the Advantages of Spinal Opioids?

Increased potency
Decreased daily dose requirements
Decreased CNS depression
Decreased incidence of ileus
Decreased potential for abuse

What Is Spinal Anesthesia?

It is a local anesthetic that is injected into the subarachnoid space, mixing with the cerebrospinal fluid (CSF) and creating conduction blockade of spinal nerves; also called *subarachnoid block*

What Are the Complications of Spinal Anesthesia?

Hypotension
Bradycardia
Cardiac arrest

Nausea and vomiting
Postdural puncture headaches

What Are the Differences Between Spinal Anesthesia and Epidural Anesthesia?

Spinal anesthesia requires that a small amount of local anesthetic be placed directly into the CSF, producing a rapid, dense, and predictable neuronal blockade. Epidural anesthesia requires an increased dose of local anesthetic in order to fill the potential epidural space and penetrate the nerve cover; for this reason, the onset is slow. The anesthesia produced is segmental in band, extending upward and downward from the injection site, and the degree of spread depends on the volume of the local anesthetic. Epidural anesthesia requires a large needle and often uses a continuous catheter. In addition, there is a subtle end-point for locating the space. The feeling of the ligaments helps locate the epidural space as the needle passes through them, whereas CSF definitively identifies the subarachnoid space.

Hemodynamic Effects of Carbon Dioxide Pneumoperitoneum (Laparoscopic) During General Anesthesia

Carbon monoxide: Decreases
Mean arterial pressure: Increases
Systemic vascular resistance: Increases
Central venous pressure: Decreases initially then increases
Pulmonary artery occlusion pressure: Initially decreases then increases

Left ventricular wall stress: Increases
Heart rate: No change

Pulmonary Changes Associated with Laparoscopy

Peak inspiratory pressure: Increased
Intrathoracic pressure: Increased
Vital capacity: Decreased
Functional residual capacity: Decreased
Respiratory compliance: Decreased
Respiratory resistance: Increased
$Paco_2$: Increased
pH: Decreased
Pao_2: No change

NOTES

Urology

David Brandli, M.D.

BENIGN RENAL TUMORS

Simple Renal Cyst

1. Most common benign renal mass lesion
2. Not true tumors but found in 50% of patients older than 50 years
3. Found more commonly with frequency of modern computed tomography (CT)
4. Smooth-walled, serum-like fluid within; universally benign unless thickened wall, complex center, or increasing size

Hyperdense Cyst

1. Smooth-walled like simple renal cyst but homogenous, hyperdense center; center often with high protein content; sometimes from hemorrhage
2. Generally does not enhance with contrast
3. Almost always benign, but warrants observation with serial imaging

Fibroma

Uncommon fibrous tumors found in renal parenchyma; can be indistinguishable from malignant tumor

Lipoma

1. Uncommon; occurs in middle-aged women
2. Many are variants of angiomyolipoma

Angiomyolipoma

1. Tumor composed of mature fat cells, smooth muscle cells, and blood vessels
2. Associated with tuberous sclerosis (adenoma sebaceum, epilepsy, and mental retardation; autosomal dominant inheritance)
   a. At least some features of tuberous sclerosis in 50% of patients with angiomyolipoma
   b. Angiomyolipoma in 80% of patients with tuberous sclerosis
3. By CT, −30 to −70 H units in tumor because of high fat content
4. Increasing size past 4 cm associated with pain or hemorrhage
5. No role for percutaneous biopsy in diagnosis
6. Treat with nephrectomy (consider partial) or embolization in setting of acute hemorrhage
7. 2% rate of conversion to renal cell carcinoma

Renal Oncocytoma

1. Composed of oncocytes; eosinophilic granular cells with fibrous capsule; characteristic central scar in tumor
2. 5% of all solid renal tumors: 5% bilateral
3. 10% incidence of oncocytoma and renal cell carcinoma in same tumor
   a. Must treat as if cancer
   b. Metastatic lesions or recurrences after nephrectomy rare

Renal Adenoma

1. Found exclusively in renal cortex
2. 20% incidence in autopsy studies

3. Association between size and malignant potential
   a. Historically, <3 cm thought to be benign
   b. Small solid renal masses should be considered malignant until proved otherwise

MALIGNANT RENAL TUMORS

Renal Cell Carcinoma

Incidence

1. 3% of adult tumors, >90% of malignant renal tumors
2. Increased risk in von Hippel–Lindau disease, acquired renal cystic disease, horseshoe kidney

Presentation

1. "Classic" triad: pain, hematuria, flank mass (only 10% of patients have the triad); other findings—weight loss, fever, hypertension, nonreducing left varicocele
2. The "great masquerader": Multiple paraneoplastic syndromes add diagnostic hurdles—hypercalcemia, erythrocytosis, amyloidosis, hepatic dysfunction (Stauffer syndrome)
3. Up to 66% of cases found incidentally by ultrasonography or CT: Because of incidental diagnosis, detected tumors are of lower stage and associated with improved survival

Diagnosis and Staging

1. Imaging
   a. Ultrasonography: lower cost and increased availability; good for differentiating cystic from solid masses

   b. CT: modality of choice; >95% accuracy in staging with increasing information about vessel status with three-dimensional reconstructions
   c. Magnetic resonance imaging: superior for imaging renal vessels and inferior vena cava in staging
2. Serum markers
   a. Elevated ferritin, erythropoietin, calcium, and renin; normochromic normocytic anemia is the most common hematologic abnormality associated with renal cell carcinoma
   b. Many molecular markers on the horizon
3. TNM staging widely accepted
   a. PT1 to PT2 tumor cutoff recently increased to 7 cm

Histologic Subtypes

1. Clear cell (75%): most common type, infiltrating and hypervascular
2. Papillary (10%): hypovascular, more often multifocal
3. Chromophobic (3%): localized growth, favorable prognosis
4. Sarcomatoid (<1%): invasive growth, poor prognosis

Treatment

1. In localized disease, nephrectomy is treatment of choice
   a. For tumors confined to capsule and <4 cm, partial nephrectomy equal to radical nephrectomy, with recurrence rate of 2% to 8%; increasing role of laparoscopy

   b. With spread to renal vein or inferior vena cava, recurrence increases to 50%
2. Metastatic disease
   a. Spread to lung (50%), bone (30%), lymph nodes (20%)
   b. Chemotherapy: no role, no benefit
   c. Radiation: role in palliation only
   d. Immunotherapy: only modest results at present
      - Interleukin (IL)-2: Food and Drug Administration (FDA) approved; 15% to 19% partial response, 10% durable response
      - Interferon-alfa: 10% to 20% response rate, rarely lasting beyond 2 years
      - Evidence for role of nephrectomy before immunotherapy

Other Malignant Renal Tumors

Sarcomas of Kidney

Most common is leiomyosarcoma (60%)

Metastatic Lesions

1. Lymphoma-lymphoblastoma most common
2. Also lung, ovarian, bowel, and breast

ADRENAL TUMORS

Cushing Syndrome

Etiology

1. Pituitary tumor (70%)
2. Adrenal tumor (20%)
3. Adrenal hyperplasia (5%)
4. Ectopic adrenocorticotropic hormone (ACTH) (5%)

Presentation

Glucocorticoid excess manifests as round face; truncal obesity; thin, friable skin; and hypertension.

Diagnosis

1. 24-hour urinary free cortisol best first study
2. Can proceed to overnight dexamethasone suppression test or AM/PM cortisol levels; plasma ACTH for localization of Cushing syndrome
3. CT first imaging study to obtain

Treatment

1. Pituitary adenoma often treated by transsphenoidal surgery
2. Adrenal tumors: treatment often dictated by size; possible approaches include intraperitoneal, extraperitoneal, and laparoscopic

Pheochromocytoma

Definition

Catecholamine-secreting tumor of neural crest origin

Presentation

1. Classic triad: headache, palpitations, sweating
2. Rule of 10%
   a. 10% extra-adrenal; often along sympathetic ganglia of the retroperitoneum
   b. 10% malignant
   c. 10% associated with multiple endocrine neoplasia
   d. 10% in pediatric population
   e. 10% bilateral

3. Both paroxysmal and sustained hypertension, also diabetes mellitus
4. Up to 40% of cases diagnosed incidentally

Diagnosis

1. Urinary metanephrines best first study
2. Plasma catecholamines
3. Clonidine suppression test used to differentiate pheochromocytoma from essential hypertension
4. CT radiographic study of choice—98% sensitivity

Treatment

1. Preoperative preparation
   a. α-Adrenergic blockade
   b. β-Blockers only for arrhythmias
   c. Generally, patients volume-contracted and must be vigorously hydrated
2. Surgical removal
   a. Multiple approaches available, including laparoscopic
   b. Must get vascular control first
   c. Hypertension significant during surgical manipulation, followed by hypotension after vascular occlusion

Primary Aldosteronism—Conn Syndrome

Characteristics

1. Adenoma in 60%, hyperplasia (usually bilateral) in 40%
2. Often occurs in younger adults with severe and refractory hypertension
3. Aldosterone hypersecretion, causing sodium retention, potassium wasting, and hypertension

Diagnosis

1. Hyperkalemia with low plasma renin activity: 24-hour urinary aldosterone secretion study during salt repletion most accurate
2. CT best initial radiographic study: adrenal venous sampling more accurate, especially for small tumors

Treatment

1. Hyperplasia treated with potassium-sparing diuretics
2. Adenomas surgically removed: multiple approaches available based on size and side of tumor

Adrenocortical Carcinoma

Characteristics

1. Symptoms based on endocrine activity: endocrine activity often mixed
2. Most tumors >6 cm by CT
3. Relatively uncommon malignant adrenal tumor

Treatment

Surgery: aggressive tumor with guarded prognosis even with low-stage disease

Bladder Cancer

Incidence and Risk Factors

1. 50,000 new cases each year: fourth highest cause of cancer death in men; rising in women

2. Population risk factors: white race, male sex, and advanced age
3. Other risk factors: smoking, occupational exposures (dyes, aromatic agents), chronic bladder irritation, infection

Presentation

1. Classically painless hematuria; also irritative voiding symptoms, pelvic mass, pain from ureteral obstruction or metastatic disease
2. Medical evaluation often delayed

Pathology

Transitional Cell Carcinoma (90%)

1. "Field change": irreversible damage induced throughout urothelium by carcinogens: leads to recurrent tumors and multifocal tumors
2. Can be superficial or invasive
3. Can be papillary (70%), sessile, or flat: carcinoma in situ, a flat high-grade transitional cell carcinoma, has increased rate of invasion and recurrence

Pathology

Squamous Cell Carcinoma (5%)

1. Caused by chronic irritation or infection: occurs in 10% of quadriplegics with chronic suprapubic tubes (usually after 10 years)
2. Generally thought to be aggressive and invasive

Adenocarcinoma (2%)

1. Located primarily at the dome and base of bladder

2. May be primary or metastatic: associated with urachus and bladder exstrophy
3. Tumor aggressive, with early invasion and decreased survival

Diagnosis

1. Initial work-up includes intravenous pyelography (IVP), cystoscopy, and urine cytologic studies.
2. If tumor is visible, anesthetic cystoscopy with biopsy is indicated.
3. Invasive tumor warrants CT of the abdomen and pelvis, chest films, and liver function tests.

Treatment

1. For superficial tumors, intravesical chemotherapies
   a. Bacille Calmette-Guérin—causes inflammatory reaction in bladder, which reduces tumor recurrence and progression
   b. Thiotepa, mitomycin-C
2. For invasive, progressive, recurrent, or multifocal tumors: cystectomy with pelvic lymphadenectomy
3. Metastatic disease carries poor prognosis: methotrexate, vinblastine, doxorubicin (Adriamycin), and cisplatin (MVAC) chemotherapy

TESTIS CANCER

Incidence and Risk Factors

1. 7500 new cases each year and 300 deaths
2. Most common neoplasm in men aged 15 to 45 years

3. Risk factors
   a. White race—rare in Asians and African Americans
   b. Cryptorchidism
      - 20 to 40 times increased risk
      - Risk also higher for the normally descended testicle
      - 10% of patients presenting with testis tumor have a history of cryptorchidism
   c. Testicular atrophy and mumps orchitis
   d. Trauma does not lead to testis cancer but does bring young men for examination, occasionally revealing disease

Presentation

1. Most cancers are discovered by the patient. There is often a delay of several months between discovery and medical evaluation.
2. The patient usually describes a painless mass, increasing in size. Pain is the presenting symptom only 10% of the time.

Tumor Types

1. 95% of germ cell origin
2. Seminoma: most common pure testis neoplasm
3. Nonseminomatous germ cell tumors: embryonal, yolk sac, teratoma, teratocarcinoma, choriocarcinoma
4. About two thirds of testis cancers mixed germ cell tumors
5. Non–germ cell tumors less common, including Leydig and Sertoli cell tumors

Evaluation

1. History and physical examination
2. Markers
   a. α-Fetoprotein
      - Elevated in yolk sac tumors, embryonal carcinoma, and teratocarcinoma
      - Has 5-day half-life
      - Half-lives of markers followed after orchiectomy to evaluate for disease outside testis
   b. β-Human chorionic gonadotropin
      - Elevated in choriocarcinoma and rarely in seminoma
      - Has 24-hour half-life
3. CT of the chest, abdomen, and pelvis
4. Radical orchiectomy: performed through an inguinal incision to avoid violation of the scrotal lymphatics (different from lymphatic drainage of the testis and cord)

Management

1. Seminoma
   a. Low-stage seminoma treated primarily with radiation
   b. High-stage seminoma treated with combination of chemotherapy and surgery for relapses
2. Nonseminomatous germ cell tumors
   a. Low-stage tumors treated with surgery or surveillance
   b. High-stage tumors treated with chemotherapy

PROSTATE CANCER

Incidence and Risk factors

1. 250,000 new cases each year, 50,000 deaths
2. 1 in 6 lifetime risk

3. Average age at diagnosis 72 years
4. Risk factors include:
   a. African American race: generally present with more advanced stage and more aggressive tumors, have higher mortality rate
   b. High-fat diets and low-fat diets may decrease testosterone levels
   c. Family history—related to age at diagnosis for affected relative

Evaluation

1. History and physical examination, including digital rectal examination
2. Transrectal ultrasound and biopsy if indicated
   a. Cancer appears hypoechoic; 85% of tumors multifocal
   b. Gleason sum pathologic score with proven prognostic significance
3. Metastatic work-up indicated if prostate-specific antigen >20 ng/dL or if symptoms significant
   a. CT of abdomen and pelvis
   b. Chest radiography
   c. Liver function tests, including alkaline phosphatase determination
   d. Bone scan indicated if alkaline phosphatase level elevated to detect bone metastasis, the most common site of hematogenous spread

Treatment

1. Must carefully consider patient life expectancy in treatment algorithm
   a. Traditionally held that patients with life expectancy <10 years should not receive aggressive treatment for prostate cancer

   b. Life expectancy estimates often flawed—for example, average life expectancy for 70-year-old man is 15 years
2. Radical prostatectomy is the gold standard for organ-confined disease.
   a. Retropubic or perineal approaches: no technique proved superior—surgeon's preference
   b. Up to 50% of clinically organ-confined tumors found to be understaged at time of surgery
   c. Pelvic lymph node dissection (most common site of lymph spread) generally performed, but nodes not analyzed by frozen section unless palpably abnormal
3. Radiation therapy: external beam or placement of interstitial seeds—multiple isotope sources: head-to-head comparison with surgery lacking
4. Hormonal deprivation—deprives prostate tumor of testosterone
   a. For advanced, metastatic, or symptomatic disease
   b. Bilateral orchiectomy or pharmacologic treatment
5. Watchful waiting

BENIGN PROSTATIC HYPERPLASIA

Characteristics

1. Characterized by bladder outlet obstruction causing increased voiding pressure with decreased urinary flow rate
2. Benign condition with far-reaching impact on medical resources

3. In one study, 50% of men older than age 60 had diagnosis of benign prostatic hyperplasia
4. Is not a precursor lesion for prostate cancer
5. Largest cause of emergency room visits for urinary retention

Signs and Symptoms

Urinary frequency and urgency, incontinence, decreased stream, hematuria, uninhibited bladder contractions, bladder stones, and renal failure

Evaluation

Evaluation is with history and physical examination, including digital rectal examination, urinary flow rate, and post-voiding residual

Treatment

1. Medical therapies include α-blockers, which reduce smooth muscle around the gland, easing voiding and androgen suppression.
2. Surgical therapies include transurethral resection of the prostate (TURP), laser therapies, thermotherapies, high-intensity focused ultrasound therapy, and various urethral stents.
   a. TURP is considered to be the gold standard.
   b. TURP syndrome results from the systemic absorption of hypotonic bladder irrigation through the prostatic venous channels with resulting hyponatremia, cerebral edema, and seizures.

UROLOGIC EMERGENCIES

Testicular Torsion

Two Types

1. Extravaginal (5%)—occurs before birth or shortly thereafter; includes twisting of cord and tunica vaginalis; common cause of undescended testis
2. Intravaginal (95%)—associated with pubertal increase of testis size as testis twists within the tunica vaginalis: 360- to 720-degree twist required to compromise blood supply

Incidence/Risk Factors

1. Risk of having acute scrotal event by age 25 years, 1 in 160
2. Average age, 12 years; left more common than right; bilateral 2%
3. Risk factors: "bell clapper deformity"—a side-ways lie of the testis in the dependent scrotum

Presentation

1. Pain (universal)
   a. Usually ends current activities
   b. Children younger than 18 years more likely to seek help quickly; those older than 18 years more likely to keep problem private as long as possible
2. Nausea and vomiting (25%)
3. Swollen, dark-red hemiscrotum, initially very tender
4. Absent cremasteric reflex
5. Children with acute scrotum often are marginally ambulatory

Evaluation

1. If history and physical examination results are unequivocal, operative correction indicated: Manual detorsion can be attempted with local anesthetic preoperatively, but this does not obviate the need for surgery.
2. Testicular ultrasound imaging/Doppler study can be used for equivocal cases, as can a nuclear medicine study, but both take valuable time.

Treatment

1. Surgical detorsion is performed through inguinal incision.
   a. Ideally, surgery is performed within 4 hours of the onset of symptoms.
   b. Infarction is certain after 16 hours of complete vessel occlusion.
2. Follow-up shows reduced sperm counts and fertility for patients after torsion even with a normal contralateral testis; this may be due to a deleterious substance from diseased testis or pathologic process that predisposed testis to torsion and affects other side.

Other Causes of Acute Scrotum

1. Acute epididymitis: The problem most likely to mimic testicular torsion. Differential diagnosis can include fever, leucocytosis, or urinary tract infection.
2. Appendiceal torsion
   a. Epididymal and testicular appendages remaining from development are pedunculated and can twist, compromising blood supply.

   b. "Blue dot" sign sometimes is visible through skin.
   c. Pain is less severe and more gradual; it can present days after onset.
   d. Treatment is with anti-inflammatory drugs and time.
3. Trauma: Always ask about trauma.

Priapism

Characteristics

1. Prolonged erection (>6 hours) not associated with sexual stimulation
2. Glans and periurethral spongiosum often soft in priapism relative to corporal bodies

Types

1. Low flow or ischemic—more common; associated with failure of corporal venous return
2. High flow or non–ischemic—associated with trauma and arterial leak; generally less painful
3. Arterial blood gases from corporeal blood can help differentiate

Etiology

1. Idiopathic (30% to 60%), sickle cell disease, trauma, alcohol-drugs, medication (trazodone), iatrogenic (intracorporeal injections for impotence)
2. Age peaks at 10 and 40 years

Treatment

1. High-flow priapism is generally treated with arteriography and embolization of the damaged vessel.

2. Low-flow priapism
    a. Conservative measures: sedation, ice-cold enemas, epidural-spinal anesthesia, ketamine
    b. Invasive measures
        - Intracorporeal clot evacuation with instillation of phenylephrine
        - Surgical shunts to take blood from corpora to spongiosum

Paraphimosis

Characteristics

1. There is an inability to return the foreskin over the glans.
2. It is often secondary to recurrent infections, trauma, and scar formation.
3. Treat with manual compression of the swollen foreskin and glans to allow foreskin to return to normal position.
4. Caretakers must always manually return the foreskin over the glans to avoid paraphimosis.
5. Phimosis, an inability to retract the foreskin, is not an emergency unless accompanied by infection or urinary retention.

Fournier Gangrene

Characteristics

1. Aggressive multiorganism infection of the genital and perineal areas causing necrosis, massive tissue loss, sepsis, and death in 50% of patients.
    a. Organisms are largely anaerobes.
    b. Predisposing conditions include diabetes, immunosuppression, and obesity.
    c. Treatment is wide, aggressive débridement and broad-spectrum antibiotics.

UROLOGIC TRAUMA

Renal Trauma

Incidence

1. All trauma more common in males aged 16 to 25 years
2. 90% of renal trauma is blunt (motor vehicle accidents, falls, sports injuries), 10% penetrating (firearm, knife)
3. Vascular injuries
   a. Artery 20%, vein 35%, both 45%
   b. Segmental arterial injury leads to segmental infarct due to lack of collateral arterial circulation in the kidney

Presentation-Evaluation

1. Significant hematuria (>5 red blood cells per high-power field) *or* gross hematuria *or* shock (systolic blood pressure <90 mm Hg) *or* clinical indication justifies clinical staging (IVP or CT).
   a. Children are an exception: any child (<16 years) with any degree of hematuria must undergo imaging.
   b. History is often less reliable; the kidney in children is relatively large and less protected, and hypotension is a later sign of serious injury in children.

Imaging Studies

1. CT: study of choice for staging renal injuries
   a. Vascular and collecting system injuries as well as those of the parenchyma can be detected with high sensitivity.
   b. CT has largely replaced angiography.

c. CT is ubiquitous in the evaluation of trauma.
d. New scanners are faster and give more detailed images.

2. Intravenous pyelography
   a. Largely replaced by CT
   b. Often used for "one-shot" IVP intraoperatively to confirm contralateral renal function
3. Arteriography: useful in confirming or delineating renal vascular injuries and in embolization therapy
4. Ultrasound imaging: limited role in defining renal injuries—gives no information about function of kidney

Grading

1. Grade I: hematuria with or without subcapsular hematoma
2. Grade II: grade I plus cortical laceration <1 cm deep
3. Grade III: grade II plus cortical laceration >1 cm deep without extravasation
4. Grade IV: grade III with extravasation or segmental arterial thrombosis
5. Grade V: multiple major lacerations or thrombosis-avulsion of the main renal vessels

Treatment

1. Grades I and II are considered minor injuries and are usually observed; grades III and IV require more clinical judgment; grade V (10% to 15% of total) usually treated with surgery
2. Trend in the literature toward more conservative approach to renal trauma; operate only when completely necessary

   a. Absolute indications for surgery: renal bleeding with shock, expanding or pulsatile hematoma in retroperitoneum, main renal artery injury bilaterally or in a solitary kidney
   b. Relative indications: nonviable tissue, urinary extravasation, renal artery thrombosis, concomitant laparotomy for associated injuries
3. Penetrating renal trauma
   a. Most are major injuries and exploration is planned for other associated injuries as well.
   b. Imaging should be obtained for any penetrating renal injury with any hematuria.
   c. Recent review of penetrating renal injuries showed that 50% were managed conservatively.
4. Vascular injuries
   a. Many occur in patients with multiple trauma, and nephrectomy is performed after contralateral function is confirmed.
   b. Most cases of segmental arterial thrombosis are treated with observation.
   c. Vascular repair
      - Arterial repair less often successful than venous
      - In one large series, arterial repair was successful in only 4 of 12 cases
      - Early repair affords best chance for salvage

Ureteral Trauma

Incidence and Presentation

1. Less than 1% of all genitourinary trauma: must have high index of suspicion
2. Several mechanisms
   a. Penetrating—relatively common

   b. Blunt—ureteral blunt trauma relatively uncommon
   c. Crush
   d. Avulsion—classic example hyperextension in children with ureteropelvic junction avulsion
   e. Iatrogenic transection or ligation—most common mechanism
3. Presentation
   a. Hematuria—absent in 25% of cases
   b. Inferred by mechanism, path of projectile, and so on

Diagnosis

1. No single imaging study reliably excludes ureteral injury.
2. Direct inspection during laparotomy is most reliable.
   a. Methylene blue can be used to better appreciate injury.
   b. Ureter can also be occluded to see leak.
3. IVP or CT is not reliable, even if contrast fills the bladder.

Management

1. Ideally, operative repair should be undertaken in less than 5 days.
   a. Beyond 5 days, repair after a delay of several months is preferred.
   b. Ureteral stenting is sometimes needed to control leak.

Principles of Ureteral Repair

1. Primary anastomosis is preferred: emphasize tension-free, spatulated water-tight anastomosis with absorbable suture over a ureteral stent.

2. Larger ureteral defects necessitate further maneuvers.
   a. Transureteroureterostomy, ureterocalicostomy, psoas hitch, and ureteral reimplantation may be indicated.
   b. Occasionally, ureteral loss is so significant as to require ureteral replacement with ileum, but this is problematic in an unprepared bowel in the trauma setting.
   c. Nephrectomy is also sometimes necessary.

Bladder Trauma

Two General Types

1. Extraperitoneal rupture: most common type (60%)
2. Intraperitoneal rupture
   a. Less common (30%)
   b. Associated with full bladder and extreme forces
3. Combined intra- and extraperitoneal rupture rare (10%)

Presentation

1. Hematuria (95% of cases), abdominal pain, urinary retention
2. 90% of extraperitoneal bladder ruptures have associated pelvic fracture; similarly, 90% of traumatic urethral disruptions have associated pelvic fracture
3. 10% of pelvic fractures have associated bladder rupture

Imaging

1. Cystogram is the gold standard.
   a. Must fill with at least 300 mL water-soluble contrast

   b. Can use CT or plain film imaging while bladder filled
   c. Cystogram with leak gives little information about degree of injury
2. IVP is inadequate for bladder injury.

Management

1. Intraperitoneal rupture
   a. Open repair mandated if intraperitoneal rupture verified
   b. Bladder decompressed for 7 to 10 postoperative days
2. Extraperitoneal rupture
   a. Conservative management with catheter drainage often successful, depending on size of defect
   b. If open repair planned for other injuries, bladder should be repaired at this opportunity
   c. Injuries involving bladder neck should be managed operatively
3. Principles of repair: Closure must be water-tight and tension-free, with absorbable suture in multiple layers with adequate drainage.

Urethral Injuries

Incidence and Mechanism

1. High association with pelvic fracture, similar to bladder rupture
2. Most commonly from blunt trauma, rarely from penetrating trauma: straddle injury of bulbous urethra most common
3. Urethral disruption can be partial or complete

Presentation

1. Blood at urethral meatus—most reliable clinical sign
2. Pelvic fracture
3. "High-riding" prostate
4. Inability to void

Imaging

1. Retrograde pyelogram is the gold standard.
   a. Slow injection of contrast material with oblique films can reveal contrast extravasation.
   b. Partial disruption allows some contrast to leak into bladder.

Management

1. Immediate catheter alignment is mandatory for bladder neck laceration, rectal laceration, or long separation between bladder and prostate.
2. Catheter alignment should be attempted by a urologist. Flexible cystoscopy is useful for catheter placement.
3. If alignment is not possible, placement of suprapubic catheter is followed by delayed primary repair in 2 to 3 months after repeat imaging.
4. Long-term complications include incontinence, stricture, and impotence.

Genital Trauma

Penis

1. Most corporeal fractures are caused by vigorous intercourse.

   a. Associated urethral injury is possible, so retrograde urethrography is performed.
   b. Immediate surgical repair is required.
2. Laceration, skin avulsion, and amputation are also possible.

Testis

1. Rupture
   a. Secondary to blunt or penetrating trauma
   b. Diagnosis confirmed with ultrasonography
   c. Immediate surgery required for salvage of testis
2. Amputation: Microvascular repair is mandated; literature reports limited success.

Scrotum

Primary repair is preferred.

Urinary Stone Disease

Incidence

1. 5% to 15% lifetime risk of urinary stones in the United States
2. Four times higher in men
3. Recurrence rate 50% in 5 years

Types of Urinary Stones

1. Calcium oxalate: most common type (60% of total); increased risk after small bowel resection
2. Calcium phosphate: associated with renal tubular acidosis

3. Struvite: magnesium-ammonium-phosphate stones associated with urinary tract infections and high urine pH
4. Cysteine: associated with errors in cysteine metabolism

Presentation

1. Pain—depends on location of stone; usually flank, groin
2. Nausea and vomiting
3. Dysuria

Evaluation

1. Radiographic studies
   a. Noncontrast CT
      - High sensitivity and specificity for urinary tract stones
      - No contrast necessary
      - High cost
      - Now available at most modern hospitals

   b. IVP
      - Lower sensitivity and specificity for urinary tract stones
      - IV contrast
      - Lower cost
2. Laboratory studies
   a. Urinalysis and urine culture
   b. Complete blood count and chemistry studies

Treatment

1. Kidney-ureteral stones
   a. Spontaneous passage: 1 to 4 mm, 75%; 4 to 6 mm, 50%; >6 mm, 20%

b. Shock-wave lithotripsy
   - For stones <1.5 cm in renal pelvis or proximal ureter
   - Minimally invasive
c. Ureteroscopy-pyeloscopy with stone disruption (e.g., shock wave, laser): for various sizes of stones, lower pole renal stones, and ureteral stones
d. Percutaneous nephrolithotomy: access through back to kidney for larger stones

2. Bladder stones
   a. Most can be treated cystoscopically.
   b. Largest stones are extracted through open procedure.

NOTES

CHAPTER 17

Neurosurgery for the General Surgeon

Patrick Connolly, M.D.

Trauma Quick Facts

CPP

Equals MAP – ICP

Scalp Lacerations

Can account for massive blood loss; repair in the Advanced Trauma Life Support protocol primary survey

Depressed Skull Fractures

Generally, surgery if >7 mm or open

Epidural Hematoma

Bilenticular shape, middle fossa, middle meningeal artery rupture

Glasgow Coma Score

Less than 8, intubate—has motor, verbal, and eye opening components; less than 8 warrants ICP monitoring after trauma

Subdural Hematoma

Crescent shape along brain surface; higher energy injury, usually comes with brain damage and edema; midline shift greater than thickness of subdural hematoma portends poor prognosis

Penetrating Head Injury

Glasgow Coma Score (GCS) of 12 to 15 = good outcome; GCS of 3 to 5 = universal death; ventricle, midline, or brain stem damage portends poor prognosis

Empirical ICP therapy for signs of a mass lesion (i.e., blown pupil, hemiparesis, hemiposturing, or Cushing reflex [bradycardia, hypertension, agonal respiration]); triad rare; any one element matter of concern

ICP Management (Treat ICP >20 mmHg)

1. Head of bed elevated 30 degrees
2. Light sedation
3. Head in midline position
4. Heavy sedation requiring intubation
5. Mannitol
6. Hyperventilation
7. Ventricular drainage
8. Barbiturate coma
9. Lobectomy or craniectomy

Who Requires ICP Monitoring?

1. Abnormal-appearing CT and GCS <8
2. Normal CT, GCS <8, and one of the following: systolic blood pressure <90 mmHg, age >40 years, or hemiposturing-hemiparesis)

Steroids

Harmful in head injury, controversial in spinal cord injury; most neurosurgeons in the United States recommend high-dose methylprednisolone

Central Cord Syndrome

Hyperextension injury
Dysesthesias more common in upper than lower extremities
Sacral sparing
Commonly overlooked in the emergency room

More Trauma Quick Facts

Anterior Cord Syndrome

Uncommon
Due to traumatic disk herniation or rupture
Motor deficit and pain, temperature deficit with preservation or vibration and proprioception

Brown-Séquard Syndrome

Uncommon
Hemicord malfunction
Ipsilateral paresis below level of lesion
Ipsilateral light and vibration loss
Contralateral pain and temperature loss

Astrocytoma

Glioblastoma subtype most common and has poorest prognosis, 9-month median survival

NEOPLASM QUICK FACTS

CNS Syndromes Featuring General Surgery Neoplasms

Syndrome	Gene/ Chromosome	Non–Central Nervous System Tumor Association
Neurofibromatosis type I	*NF1*/17q11	Pheochromocytoma
von Hippel–Lindau disease	*VHL*/3p25	Pheochromocytoma, renal cell carcinoma
Tuberous sclerosis	*TSC1*/9q34 *TSC2*/16p13	Cardiac rhabdomyoma, adenomatous polyps of small bowel
Li-Fraumeni syndrome	*TP53*/17p13	Breast, adrenal cancer, sarcomas
Lhermitte–Duclos syndrome	*PTEN*/10q23	Colon polyps, breast cancer, thyroid
Turcot syndrome	Numerous	Colon polyps

Meningioma

Arises from arachnoid, commonly calcified, usually enhances, may have surrounding parenchymal edema. Benign, but may recur, particularly in skull base locations where safe total resection is not possible.

Metastases

Lung, breast, renal cell, testis, and skin most common; resection of accessible solitary lesion has survival benefit, independent of tumor type

Pituitary

1. Functional adenomas most common (80%)
   a. Prolactin
   b. Growth hormone
   c. Adrenocorticotropic hormone
2. Malignant <1% of cases
3. Occasional presentation (1%) with apoplexy—severe headache, visual loss, acute addisonian crisis

Ring Enhancing Lesion

Metastasis, abscess, glioma, infarct (late), contusion (late), dermoid tumor, radiation necrosis

PEDIATRIC NEUROSURGERY QUICK FACTS

Hydrocephalus

About 1 in 1500 births
Half occur in premature babies
Ventriculoperitoneal shunting primary treatment; other options include V-pleural, V-atrial, V-gallbladder
Revision required in 40% of patients in first year after placement

Germinal Matrix Hemorrhage

45% of newborns <1500 g
Associated with hypoxia
Signs of increased ICP or progressive head growth warrant diversion of CSF

Myelomeningocele

This open neural tube defect is the most severe form of spinal dysraphism.
Incidence is about 0.7 per 1000 births, higher in the British Isles.
Folate supplementation significantly reduces incidence.
Most patients have Chiari II malformation, a minority are symptomatic.
A ventriculoperitoneal shunt is required in 90%.
Tethered cord syndrome results from adhesion of spinal cord to dura. It presents with the constellation of back pain, urinary retention-incontinence, lower extremity weakness, or progressive scoliosis.

Spinal Dysraphism

May be associated with complex urogenital malformations (e.g., myelocystocele)
Ranges from spina bifida occulta to meningocele to meningomyelocele

Craniosynostosis

It occurs in about 1 per 2000 births.
The occurrence may be isolated or syndromic.
A sagittal location is most common and it is most frequently nonsyndromic.
Occipital plagiocephaly more commonly results from head position (think of a flat basketball), not lambdoid synostosis.
Crouzon and Apert syndromes are craniofacial dysmorphic disorders (incidence, 1:25,000 and 1:55,000, respectively).

VASCULAR NEUROSURGERY QUICK FACTS

Cerebral Blood Flow

Normal = 50 mL/100 g/min
Ion gradient breakdown and cell death occur at <15 mL/100 g/min

Stroke

Third leading cause of death in the United States behind heart disease and cancer
Two types: *ischemic* (embolic or thrombotic) and *hemorrhagic* (intracerebral or subarachnoid)
Prevention most effective method to reduce incidence

Preictal Diagnosis and Risk Stratification

Duplex ultrasonography of carotid arteries identifies patients at risk. Concordant magnetic resonance angiography or plain angiography increases diagnostic accuracy. Ultrasound imaging alone misidentifies many patients as candidates or noncandidates for surgery.
Patients suffering a transient ischemic attack or other symptoms and with >50% stenosis may benefit from carotid endarterectomy. Patients with stenosis >60% and who are asymptomatic may benefit from carotid endarterectomy. Medical management (platelet antiaggregants) is superior in cases of less stenosis.

Treatment of atrial fibrillation with anticoagulation reduces the risk of cardiogenic embolus 20-fold. Aspirin is also an option.

Treatment of Stroke

Airway, breathing, circulation
Head CT
If systolic blood pressure is >160, reduce gently. Use tissue plasminogen activator if indicated. Treat atrial fibrillation. Aggressively manage hyperglycemia. Institute rehabilitation.

Saccular Aneurysm

Annual incidence of subarachnoid hemorrhage is 10:100,000. The prevalence of aneurysm is much higher. Treatment of unruptured aneurysms remains controversial (>10 mm, generally indicated).

Subarachnoid Hemorrhage

Severe apoplectic headache, stiff neck, photophobia, vomiting
ICP may be increased in relation to hydrocephalus or mass lesion; head CT 98% sensitive in first 24 hours
Dilantin, nimodipine, isotonic fluids, ventriculostomy, arterial line monitoring, emergent angiography
Aneurysmal rehemorrhage rate 4% in the first 24 hours, with 50% mortality rate; endovascular methods rapidly evolving; gold standard direct obliteration within first 72 hours.

Intracerebral Hemorrhage

Initial management is similar to that for ischemic stroke but for reverse anticoagulation. Surgery can help for patients with a depressed level of consciousness or a medium-sized clot in the basal ganglia and who are not moribund.

NOTES

Otolaryngology (Ear, Nose, Throat)

William Hoffman, M.D.

ENT FOR SURGEONS: THYROID

What Is the Basic Work-Up of the Thyroid Nodule?

1. History and physical examination
2. Fine-needle aspiration
3. Iodine-131 examination

What Is the Most Common Benign Tumor of the Thyroid Gland?

The adenoma; it concentrates iodine, and so appears "hot" on scan. Occasionally, it may bleed and become acutely painful. Thyrotoxicosis can occur if the adenoma becomes autonomous, but this is generally a late development.

What Is the Most Common Malignant Tumor? In Addition, What Are the Other Three Malignancies?

The most common malignant tumor is the papillary tumor. It is notable for lymphatic metastasis, multifocal disease in the gland, and propensity for local spread. Distant metastases are rare. The other types are follicular (hematogenous metastasis), medullary (associated with multiple endocrine neoplasia [MEN]), and anaplastic (almost routinely fatal).

Name the Risk Factors for Malignancy.

1. Rapid growth of nodule
2. Age <20 or >60 years
3. History of irradiation of the neck
4. Male gender
5. Family history of medullary thyroid carcinoma

Name Some of the Common Signs of Malignancy.

1. Hoarseness and pain
2. A hard nodule
3. A fixed nodule

What Is Werner Syndrome?

MEN-1, which includes hyperparathyroidism, pancreatic islet cell tumors, carcinoid of the stomach, and pituitary tumors. The thyroid is not involved, in contrast to the other MEN syndromes.

What Is Sipple Syndrome?

MEN-2A, which includes medullary carcinoma of the thyroid, pheochromocytoma, and hyperparathyroidism. If this entity is diagnosed, all family members should be evaluated. MEN-2B is also recognized and involves medullary carcinoma, pheochromocytoma, mucosal neuromas, and a marfanoid habitus.

What Are the Main Risks of Thyroid Surgery?

The most worrisome are bleeding and damage to the recurrent laryngeal nerve. Per gram, the thyroid is the most vascular organ of the body, and bleeding can be extensive. The recurrent nerve is generally in a predictable location, with the inferior thyroid artery being the best landmark. However, the nerve may be nonrecurrent (about 1 in 200 cases).

When Should Hyperthyroidism Be Treated Surgically?

Thyroidectomy should be performed only when the patient is euthyroid. Consider suppression with iodine and blood pressure control with propranolol.

What Is the Most Common Form of Hyperthyroidism?

Graves disease; in elderly adults, Plummer disease (nodular toxic goiter) is more common.

TUMORS OF THE SALIVARY GLANDS

What Are the Most Common Benign Tumors of the Salivary Glands?

Most common is the pleomorphic adenoma, followed by the Warthin tumor (oncocytoma); Warthin tumors may be bilateral.

What Are the Most Common Malignant Tumors of the Salivary Glands?

The most common is mucoepidermoid carcinoma, followed by adenoid cystic carcinoma. Less common are adenocarcinomas. The best test to evaluate the lesion is fine-needle aspiration.

What Is the Treatment of Salivary Gland Tumors?

Treatment is generally wide local excision of the tumor. In the parotid gland, this is best accomplished by superficial parotidectomy with dissection of the facial nerve. Tumors should not be simply shelled out because the risk of recurrence in that situation is generally >40%. Even though most tumors are benign, all should be excised because of the possibility of malignant degeneration.

What Needs to Be Considered in Adenoid Cystic Carcinoma?

Nerve involvement; this form has a propensity for nerve invasion, with skip lesions in the nerve being common. This is the main reason for the high recurrence rate with adenoid cystic disease.

What About Salivary Gland Tumors in Children?

The most common salivary gland tumor in children is still the pleomorphic adenoma. This is followed by benign hemangioma and well-differentiated mucoepidermoid.

What Are Common Signs of Malignancy?

Sudden growth of the mass
Pain
Facial nerve paralysis or paresthesias in other nerve distributions

What Is the Prognosis of Salivary Gland Malignancy?

The prognosis is generally good, as most of these tumors can be caught early because of their locations. However, if metastatic disease is present, survival is greatly reduced.

What Is Frey Syndrome?

It is gustatory sweating due to innervation of sweat glands by the postganglionic parasympathetic fibers. This is common after parotidectomy but may occur after any salivary gland excision.

A Man Presents with Markedly Enlarged Cystic Parotid Glands. He Is HIV-Positive. Is This Situation a Cause for Concern?

Not at all. This situation most likely represents benign lymphoepithelial lesions in the parotid gland. The treatment is aspiration if the lesions are grossly enlarged and treatment with the HIV "cocktail."

Name the Branches of the Facial Nerve.

Going from superior to inferior:

1. Temporal
2. Zygomatic

3. Buccal
4. Marginal mandibular
5. Cervical

The first two branches make up the upper division, the last three the lower. The divisions take off at the pes anserinus. The nerve shows considerable variability.

What Gland Is Most Often Occluded?

Submandibular gland. The stone occluding the duct is usually hydroxyapatite. The parotid gland may also become obstructed, but these stones tend to be radiolucent.

BONY TRAUMA

Temporal Bone

What Are the Two Main Types of Temporal Bone Fractures?

1. The first type is longitudinal. Fractures tend to follow the long axis of the petrous pyramid. They tend to result from lateral blunt trauma. The cochlea is generally spared, but hearing loss may result from ossicular damage.
2. The second type is transverse. The fracture generally crosses the petrous pyramid, with the fracture line often involving the foramen magnum. This often disrupts the otic capsule and leads to sensorineural hearing loss.
3. Of these two types, the longitudinal fracture is most common.

When Would a Temporal Bone Fracture Be Considered an Emergency?

When the facial nerve is paralyzed. The patient may require decompression or at least the administration of IV steroids.

When Is Facial Nerve Paralysis Most Likely? Is This the Most Common Cause?

The most likely fracture to cause paralysis is a transverse fracture. However, given that the vast majority of fractures are longitudinal, the most likely cause of traumatic facial paralysis is a longitudinal fracture.

What Are the Common Signs of Temporal Bone Fracture?

1. Battle's sign—ecchymosis of the mastoid
2. Blood behind the eardrum
3. Ear canal laceration
4. Hearing loss or vertigo, or both

Bony Facial Trauma

What Is a Tripod Fracture?

It is disruption of the zygoma in at least three places. Classically, the locations are the zygomaticofrontal suture, the arch, and the zygomaticomaxillary suture. The result is a free-floating piece of bone. Orbital and maxillary sinus fractures should be evaluated in the presence of a tripod fracture.

Describe the LeFort I Procedure.

Essentially, the maxilla is dissociated at the level of the dentition. Teeth move on examination. The remainder of the midface is stable.

Describe the LeFort II Procedure.

This is more of a pyramidal dissociation. Fracture lines extend from the nasofrontal sutures through the medial wall and floor of the orbit, and then through the pterygoid plates. The nose and maxilla move in relation to the remainder of the midface.

Describe the LeFort III Fracture (alias, *the Big Crunch*).

Damage is similar to the LeFort II fracture but also includes separation of the zygomaticofrontal suture line. The entire midface moves in relation to the eyes.

When Should These Be Repaired?

This is controversial. Most surgeons repair the fractures in 7 to 10 days, thereby allowing much of the edema to settle. Some still argue for early reduction to take advantage of the relative ease in reducing the fractures.

Other Concerns in Severe Facial Trauma

1. CSF leaks may occur with LeFort II and III fractures.
2. Injury to the globe should be ruled out.

3. Malocclusion is possible. If necessary, the patient can be placed in intermaxillary fixation (IMF).

SOFT TISSUE TRAUMA

What Are the Trauma Zones of the Neck?

They move from inferior to superior:

1. Zone I extends from the clavicle to the inferior edge of the cricoid cartilage. Injuries here are associated with high morbidity and mortality.
2. Zone II extends from the lower border of the cricoid to the angle of the mandible. Injuries here are associated with a better prognosis.
3. Zone III extends from the angle of the mandible to the skull base. Exposure here is difficult, and consequently injuries here carry a poor prognosis.

How Is Neck Trauma Best Managed?

This is an area of controversy. Some still argue that any wound traversing the platysma in zone II mandates surgical exploration and that any wound in the other zones merits angiography. Most others would argue that if the patient is stable, neck wounds can be treated conservatively. Any neck wound in the setting of hemodynamic instability warrants exploration. Angiography remains the gold standard for evaluation of the great vessels of the neck.

When Should Esophageal Injury Be Suspected?

Investigate for esophageal injury when the patient complains of severe pain on swallowing or cannot swallow secretions. The pattern of injury may also raise suspicion of injury. Gastrografin esophagography or operative endoscopy can be used to evaluate the injury.

When Should Laryngeal Trauma Be Suspected?

Bruising over the larynx may suggest trauma. Crepitation in the neck is another strong sign. Fine-cut CT shows such injuries. Patients should undergo intubation immediately and definitive repair of the fractures within a week.

COMMON EAR-NOSE-THROAT PROBLEMS IN THE INTENSIVE CARE UNIT

What Is the Basic Treatment of Sinusitis?

1. Remove all tubes from the nose (e.g., naso-gastric, airway).
2. Use decongestants (oxymetazoline [Afrin] nasal spray for 3 days).
3. Consider a nasal steroid to relieve inflammation.

Are Sinus Punctures Useful for Diagnosis?

These are useful only if pus is obtained. After a period of antibiotic therapy, pus is a rare finding. Some would argue that punctures are useless and that a swab of matter from the middle meatus is more beneficial.

How Are Nosebleeds Best Handled?

As a rule, they are best handled with as little intervention as possible. Minor nosebleeds generally stop with pressure or oxymetazoline spray, or both. A strong posterior bleed requires an anteroposterior pack. If the bleed is uncontrollable with packing, embolization is an excellent option as opposed to ligation or embolization of terminal branches of the maxillary artery and ethmoid artery.

NOTES

Miscellaneous

Rafael Azuaje, M.D.

First Muscle to Recover from General Anesthesia

Diaphragm

Most Important Cell that Produces Nitric Oxide

Macrophage

IL-1 (Macrophages)

Lymphocyte activation

IL-2 (T-Lymphocyte)

T-cell proliferation
B-cell function

IL-2b

Improves disease-free survival in patients with metastatic melanoma.

IL-6 (Monocyte)

Hepatic acute-phase response
B-cell differentiation factor

IL-10 (T Lymphocytes and Macrophages)

Inhibits macrophages
Suppresses inflammatory cytokines
Downregulator

Second Messenger for Nitric Oxide

Cyclic guanosine monophosphate (cGMP)

Inducers of Inducible Nitric Oxide Synthase (iNOS)

Endotoxin lipopolysaccharide
IL-1
Interferon-γ

Strongest Layer in a Bowel Anastomosis

Submucosa

When Intraluminal Pressure Is Increased in the Intestines, Which Pressure Increases First?

Lymphatic followed by venous and then arterial

Most Common Site of Pathologic Fracture

Humerus

Narrowest Part of the Digestive Tract

Upper esophageal sphincter

Afferent Loop Syndrome

More common after Billroth-II anastomosis

Blood Supply to Adrenal Glands

Multiple: aorta, phrenic artery, and renal artery

Chylothorax

First try conservative treatment (diets with no fats with medium-chain triglycerides, chest tube drainage, and hyperalimentation). If this fails, the thoracic duct should be ligated at its entrance to the chest via a *right* thoracotomy.

SVO_2 (Mixed Venous Oxygen)

Normal value: 66% to 77%
Less than 66%: decrease CO, decrease SaO_2
More than 77%: sepsis, cyanide poisoning, cirrhosis
SVO_2 decreases very early after a fall in CO

Most Common Cause of Increased Calcium in the United States

Malignancy

The La Place Law

$$T = \frac{1}{2} P \times R$$

Tension is directly proportional to radius; this is why the cecum is the most common site of colonic rupture (its large diameter).

The Poiseuille Law

Pressure gradient along a tube is directly proportional to the volume of flow, tube length, and fluid viscosity and is inversely proportional to the fourth power of the radius.

Causes of Nosocomial Blood Systemic Infections

1. Coagulase-negative *Staphylococcus:* 28%
2. *Staphylococcus aureus:* 16%
3. *Enterococcus:* 9%
4. *Candida:* 8%

P(A-a)O_2 (Alveolar-Arterial Oxygen Tension Difference)

Early indicator of respiratory failure
Increases in adult respiratory distress syndrome, right-to-left shunt, and hyperthermia

Pulse Oximeter Measures

Sao_2 (hemoglobin saturation of oxygen)

Auto PEEP

Usually due to gas trapping at the end of expiration (i.e., chronic obstructive pulmonary disease)
Treatment: longer endotracheal tube, prolongation of expiratory time, decreased respiratory rate and tidal volume (TV)

Normal Urine Output (Adults)

0.5 to 1 mL/kg/hr

Electrolyte Contents of Various Fluids

Source	Na	K	Cl	HCO_3
Stomach	60	15–20	140–180	0
Small Intestine	140	10	100	50
Bile	140	10	100	50
Pancreas	140	10	60–75	100
Colon	25–60	20–70	15–60	30–50
Normal saline	154	0	154	0
1/2 Normal saline	77	0	77	0
1/4 Normal saline	38.5	0	38.5	0
Ringer's lactate	130	4	110	3–28

Calculated Serum Osmolarity

$$\text{Osmolarity} = 2\text{Na} + (\text{glu}/18) + (\text{blood urea nitrogen} \div 2.8)$$

Normal value = 285 to 295 mOsm/L

Parkland Formula (Burns)

$$\text{Vol (LR)} = \text{BSA\%} \times \text{weight (kg)} \times 4$$

Give one half of volume in first 8 hours; give the rest in the next 16 hours.

Fluids

60% total body weight
- 40% of weight is intracellular fluid
- 20% of weight is extracellular fluid
  - 15% interstitial
  - 5% plasma

Adult Normal Losses

Urine, 800 to 1000 mL/day
Sweat and lungs, 750 to 1000 mL/day

Corrected Serum Calcium (Ca)

Ca = 0.8 (normal alb – patient's alb) + patient's Ca

Hypovolemia

Class I: 10% to 15% normal vs. anxious
Class II: 15% to 30% increased heart rate, pulse pressure narrowed, blood pressure okay, and urine output decreased
Class III: 30% to 40% decreased blood pressure
Class IV: >40% lethargic, coma

Normal Caloric Requirements

25 to 35 kcal/kg/day (adults)
Moderate stress 35 to 40 kcal/kg/day; severe stress 40 to 45 kcal/kg/day

Fever and Energy

Energy requirements should increase 12% with each degree of fever greater than 37°C

Protein Requirements

Maintenance: 0.8 to 1.0 g/kg/day of ideal body weight (IBW)
Repletion: up to 1.5 g/kg/day of IBW
Liver failure: 0.5 g/kg/day of IBW

Fact

Total parenteral nutrition is usually required for small bowel resection leaving less than 100 cm. Replace vitamin B_{12} when terminal ileum is resected.

RQ (Respiratory Quotient)—Volume of Carbon Dioxide Produced/Volume of Oxygen Consumed

0.6 to 0.7 fat primary fuel
0.80 to 0.85 mixed fuel sources (ideal)
More than one lipogenesis (patient receiving excessive glucose and carbohydrates being burned as fuel, risk of fatty liver and liver failure; decrease carbohydrates on hyperalimentation)
Brain's RQ 0.97 to 0.99
Starvation RQ 0.7

Refeeding Syndrome with Total Parenteral Nutrition

This occurs when a malnourished patient with decreased potassium, phosphorus, and magnesium levels is given glucose.

Half-Life of Albumin

21 days

NOTES

Index

Note: Page numbers followed by the letter t refer to tables.

B

C

D

E

F

G

H

I

K

L

M

N

O

P

Q

R

S

T

U

V